color me confident

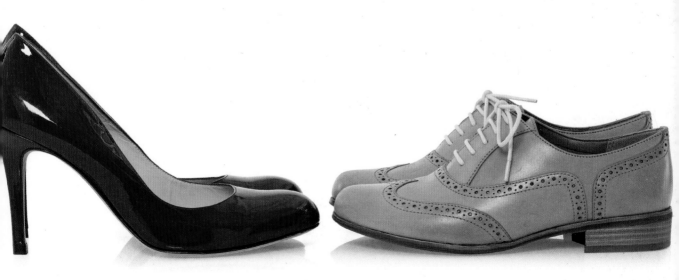

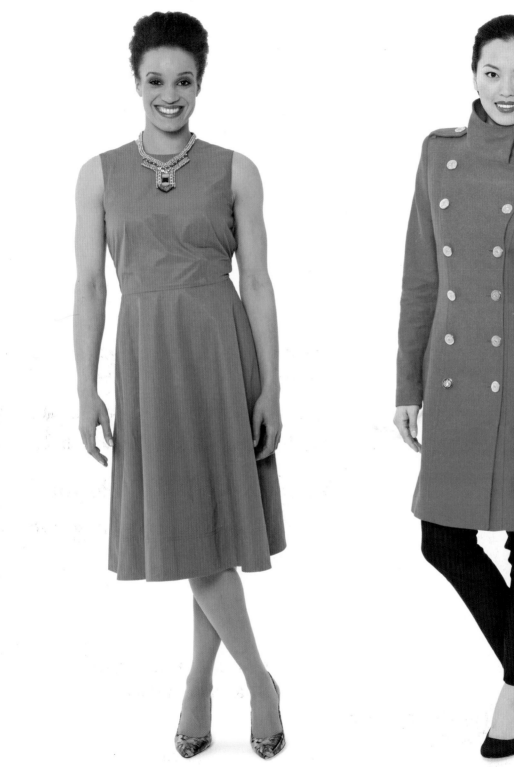

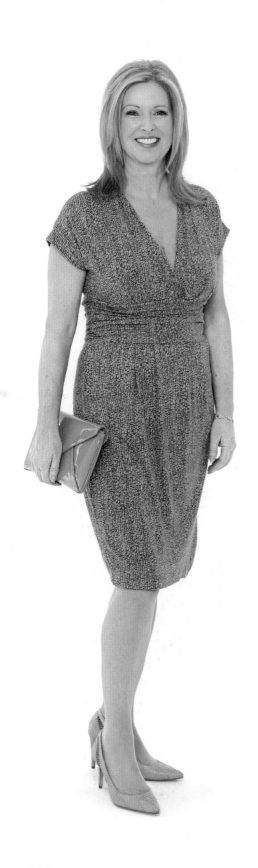

colour**me**beautiful
the image consultants

color me confident

Expert guidance to help you
look **wonderful** and feel **great**

Veronique Henderson
& Pat Henshaw

hamlyn

Dedication

To all **colour me beautiful** consultants and stylists
wherever they are in the world. Thank you for sharing your
local knowledge, inspiration, elegance, know-how, and support.
Pat & Veronique

An Hachette UK Company
www.hachette.co.uk

First published in Great Britain in 2006 by
Hamlyn, a division of Octopus Publishing Group Ltd
Endeavour House, 189 Shaftesbury Avenue
London, WC2H 8JY
www.octopusbooksusa.com

Revised and updated 2010
This revised and updated edition 2014

Distributed in the US by Hachette Book Group USA
237 Park Avenue, New York NY 10017 USA

Distributed in Canada byCanadian Manda Group
165 Dufferin Street, Toronto, Ontario, Canada M6K 3H6

ISBN 978-0-600-62818-7

Printed and bound in China

10 9 8 7 6 5 4 3 2 1

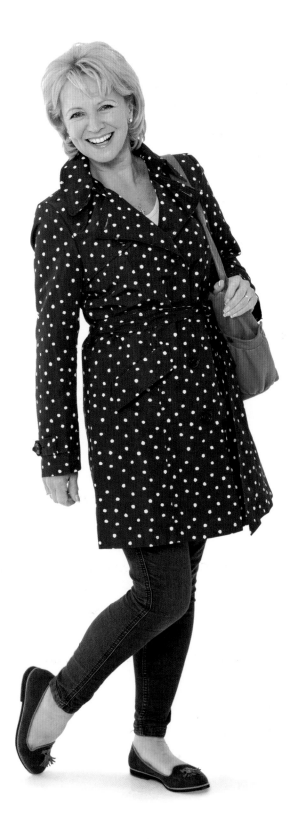

CONTENTS

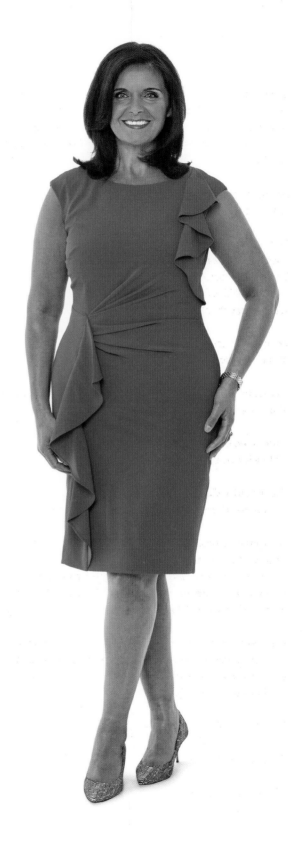

INTRODUCTION

Of the many ways in which we choose to express ourselves, the color and style of our clothes probably make the most immediate and powerful impact. Clothes do not simply cover the body and protect us from the elements—they make a visual statement about how we view ourselves. Clothes reinforce our self-image and help to define who we are. They can boost our confidence when we know we look good, but when we get it wrong, they can sap that confidence just as quickly.

Managing your appearance is an important part of who you are. It tells people about your personality and your lifestyle. Nobody can deny that, in today's world, image matters. We are bombarded with perfect images of actresses and models, and more and more emphasis is placed upon looking the part and dressing for success. We all make quick assessments based on how people look. And, while making a judgment on limited information is not the best way to go, it is important to acknowledge that clothing and personal appearance are a form of communication.

Being well dressed does not have to mean dressing expensively or being at the cutting edge of fashion. According to **colour me beautiful**, there are five key points that define a well-dressed woman. Your clothes should:

- Match your style personality
- Complement your coloring
- Flatter your body lines, scale, and proportions
- Be appropriate
- Look current

Whatever your budget, the fashion choices are endless. Increased choice can be exciting, but it can also be overwhelming and confusing. The key is to know and understand why some pieces work better than others. Forget those fashion faux pas languishing in your

closet and look forward to understanding what is special about you.

Clothes are wonderful tools that you can manipulate to your advantage, regardless of your size and proportions. By recognizing your physical assets—and limitations—you can explore the many ways in which clothing can be used to draw attention, to conceal, to camouflage, and to create optical illusions. In addition, we are all individuals with a personal style that governs the way we wear our hair, apply makeup, and tie a scarf around our neck.

ALL ABOUT COLOUR ME BEAUTIFUL

For more than 30 years **colour me beautiful** has been the world's expert in image consulting. Millions of women, and men, around the world have benefited from "having their colors done." Styling and personal image advice have become as important as being color analyzed. Over the past decade we have been commissioned to share our expertise and to this end have written seven books, which have been translated into many languages.

The company continues to develop and refine its advice from the original and simple "four seasons" approach to color to a more sophisticated system that encompasses every aspect of your personal image. While color will always be a central theme, it is only one part in

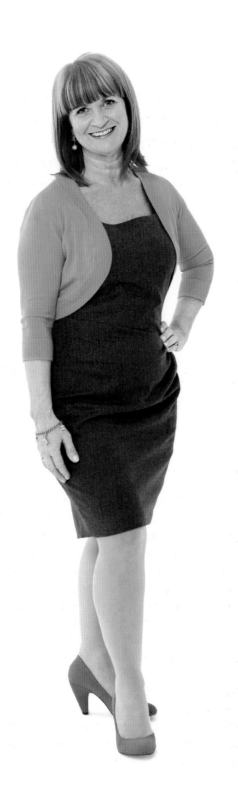

developing a personal image and style. You can enjoy taking a fresh look at how to wear colors, rather than simply learning what colors you should wear. This latest edition of our first book shows how women of all skin tones can wear color to make the most of themselves—something we believe has not been done before.

The consultants at **colour me beautiful**, some of whom are featured in this book, come from all walks of life. Many had other careers before they trained with the organization. They bring with them their collective experiences, which is what makes **colour me beautiful** the world's largest and most successful image consultancy. Other women featured in this book have experienced the **colour me beautiful** concept for the first time. They all have one thing in common—they are now confident women.

In addition to working with real women all over the world, **colour me beautiful** has developed programs for clothes stores because personal shopping is now a popular service for many small and large retailers. We also work within commerce and industry on the importance of image in business; we even help members of the motor trade sell cars to women. In recent years many consumer-goods companies have seen the benefit of adding the services of **colour me beautiful** to their promotional campaigns.

Not a day goes by without a call to the London headquarters from the national media, TV, or radio requesting information on color, image, and fashion. The questions are varied: Will this new color work for a world-class soccer team? What do you make of this movie star's shoes? So, when it comes to color, style, makeup, and staying current, you are undoubtedly in the best hands possible.

WHY READ THIS BOOK?

The aim of this book is to help you to identify the best colors for you to wear and to acknowledge your body lines, scale, and proportions. Armed with this knowledge, together with a sense of your "style personality," you will have the confidence to build a wardrobe that is practical, professional, and/or as glamorous as you need it to be. You will learn that, to meet the demands of your lifestyle, your wardrobe does not have to bulge; it just needs balance. It will become easy for you to shop efficiently, to avoid disaster purchases, and to enjoy yourself more in the whole process. Basically, you want a wardrobe that works for you. There are many demands on our lives and having clothes suitable for all occasions can often be beyond our budget and against our inclinations.

A coordinated wardrobe takes a little planning, forethought, and a strong will to avoid impulse buys. Following the guidelines given in this book will keep you on the straight and narrow without taking the fun out of shopping (for those of you who enjoy it) and without making it a torment (for those who don't). The right selection of clothes will not only make you look great physically but will also help you to feel good about yourself—and therefore you will become more confident. Wearing the right colors and flattering styles can put a smile on your face, lift your spirits, and improve your outlook.

HOW DOES THIS BOOK WORK?

This book is not about changing your physical appearance (though sometimes a little exercise and diet might help). It will not recommend liposuction, botox, or any sort of surgery. The aim is to bring out the best in you, just as the team of **colour me beautiful** consultants around the world have done every day over the past 30 years for millions of happy, confident women from all walks of life.

Does your lifestyle allow you the time and budget to visit the hairdresser twice a week? Can you spend a fortune on clothes? Do you have endless time to go shopping for clothes while juggling a full-time job, children, a partner, a dog, a garden, and a social life? In this book you will get hints and tips on how to make the most of yourself with minimal effort and budget. You may be surprised how often a shorter hemline can transform your silhouette; or maybe how some new, frivolous accessories will update a long-forgotten dress.

We start this book by looking at your unique styling personality, which in many ways will dictate your choice of styles and colors. Then we guide you to your dominant palette—be it Light, Deep, Warm, Cool, Clear, or Soft. Within each dominant category we show the different alternatives available. With Lights we will look at what can happen with the ageing process, and with all the other dominants we show you how different skin tones and coloring types can share the same color description. Armed with your palette of colors you are encouraged to assess and learn about your body, its shape and proportions, and then to choose and build your wardrobe with confidence. We will also look at various lifestyles and the working wardrobe to ensure you are always appropriately dressed for all occasions.

WHY SHOULD I USE THIS BOOK?
It will give you confidence

- By adapting your look, staying current, and developing your own individual style, you will feel more confident.
- Wearing the right color and style of clothes will make you look younger and healthier.
- Knowing how to adapt your wardrobe for different lifestyles increases your self-esteem (as well as making the most of your purchases).

It will make you unique

Your unique style—the way you wear your hair, your clothes, and how they reflect your lifestyle—is dictated by your personality. With the help of **colour me beautiful**, you will stay the same you—but become more confident. No two women will have exactly the same coloring, size, and shape, scale and proportions, personality, or budget. But it's useful to have some guidelines to help you make sense of all the choices available, and focus on what you really need.

It will help you make the most of your shape

All women wish for the perfect body but, unfortunately, nature is not always as kind as we would like. With some simple tricks and tips from **colour me beautiful** any woman can improve her appearance regardless of the size she is.

It will help you shop successfully

With so many demands on our lives, having suitable clothes for every occasion can often be beyond our reach. With a little forethought and some willpower, you will learn to avoid impulse and unwise buys, and have a wardrobe that works all year round. The days of a wardrobe full of clothes but nothing to wear will be gone. Learn the secrets that **colour me beautiful** clients discover every day in consultants' studios.

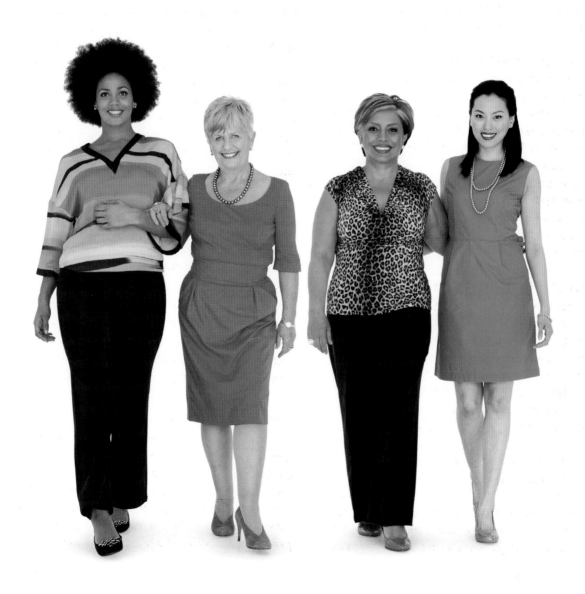

HOW TO USE THIS BOOK

You are not going to change your look in an instant. Instead, you will find that you will use this book as a manual that you will dive into over a period of time. Once you have identified your priorities from the questionnaire on the following pages, make one of them your starting point. Take it step by step and be confident with each stage—color, makeup, style, and accessories. Often, **colour me beautiful** clients will attend a color session and then come back a month later for the style session. Revisiting a concept will give you a fuller understanding and the confidence to go ahead and use your newfound insight.

There is no miracle solution. While there are some easy tips that will give instant answers, you may need time to take other advice on board. In all cases you have to start with your existing wardrobe—a tweak here and there may be all that is needed—and what your budget allows. Your ultimate aim is to become a confident person who knows how to make the most of herself and who will not hesitate to make a choice when facing her wardrobe every morning.

With sound advice for real women, backed by years of experience from the top **colour me beautiful** team, this book will show you how to achieve the head-to-toe makeover that will give you confidence and change your life. It's up to you now.

MAKING A CHANGE

Step 1 – decision time
- Identify the need for change.
- Prepare yourself for a challenge.

Step 2 – style personality
- Identify your style personality and learn how to enhance it: go to pages 22–37.

Step 3 – color
- By understanding how color is made up, you will see how colors look together and work best to flatter you: go to pages 40–49.
- Color makes the initial impact, so find out what colors will be perfect for you. See Chapter 4, Your color type (pages 50–115).
- Read about the science of color to understand that although you will have 36 recommended colors, these, in fact, represent thousands of colors that you can wear: go to pages 112–113.

Step 4 – style
- Take a long look at yourself to establish your basic body shape: go to pages 118–123.
- From your neck to your ankles, analyze every detail of your body: go to page 120.
- Learn which fabrics and textures flatter your body shape: go to pages 124–135.
- Scale and proportions matter too—and this book shows you why: go to pages 136–139.

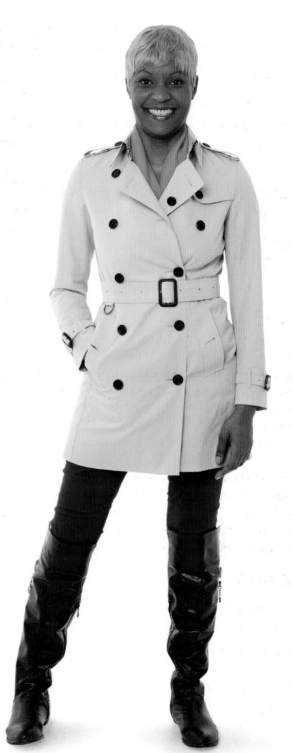

Step 5 – shopping habits

• Learn how to shop effectively for clothes that look good on you and go together, thus creating a versatile wardrobe: go to pages 170–177.

• Whether the thought of shopping leaves you cold or you come to life in the shopping mall, you can learn to use shopping time wisely and to shop efficiently within your budget: go to page 198–199

Step 6 – putting it into action

• Pulling it all together: styling personality + color + body shape + scale + proportions + accessories + budget = the real you.

Once you know you look good, you are ready to face the world— or any situation that calls for poise and control

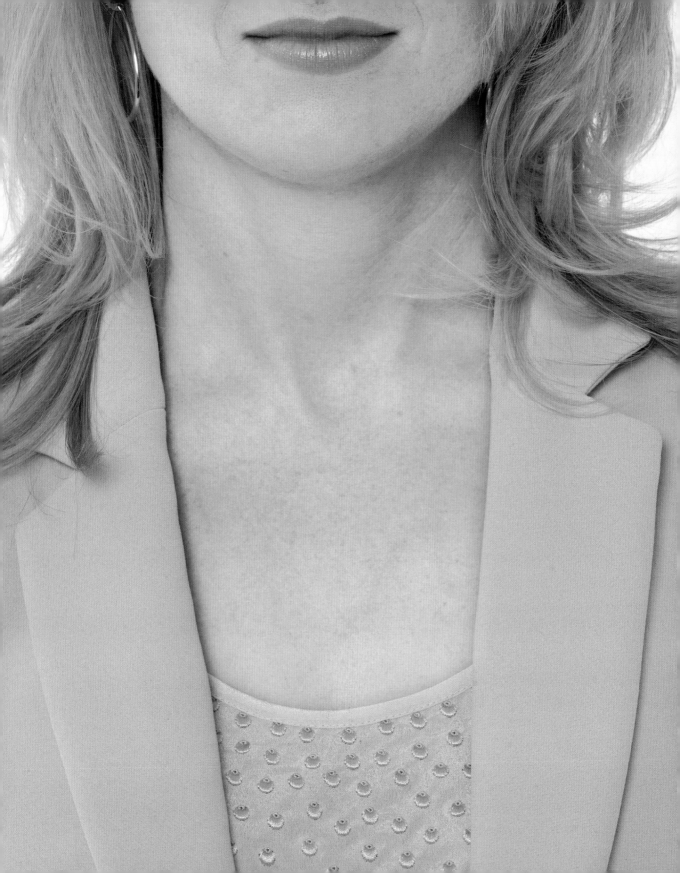

1

TIME FOR A CHANGE

TAKE A FRESH LOOK

For whatever reason—perhaps a new job, your children leaving home, or meeting a new partner—there are periods in every woman's life when the clothes that always seemed right just don't do the job anymore. This is the time to take a fresh look at yourself and to take steps to develop a style that is uniquely your own.

Every day you meet new people, and some of them may become friends, even foes. Do you feel confident when you meet someone for the first time? Only 7 percent of a person's judgment of you is based on what you say to them. The rest of their judgment is based on your appearance and body language. So, when you are getting ready to meet new people, do you know exactly what to wear, or do you end up with a pile of clothes on the bedroom floor and emerge wearing your old favorites? Try this confidence test:

THE CONFIDENCE TEST

Stand (fully dressed) in front of the mirror, then:

1 Look at yourself

2 Smile

3 Pay yourself a compliment

If you find this easy to do, then congratulations. It is more likely, however, that you will have found only faults: that you're not tall enough/your legs are too short/your hair is lifeless. But how many women who wish for longer legs actually have wonderfully long bodies? Likewise, some women may complain that their waists are too big, even though they invariably have small bottoms and hips. This book will help you start to look at yourself in a new, more positive way. We would like to help you to identify your best features and learn to disregard the parts of your body that you are unsure about.

PLANNING FOR THE FUTURE

Most women wear only 20 percent of their wardrobe 80 percent of the time. Matching your wardrobe to your lifestyle takes a little thought and time, but once you get to grips with it you will always have something to wear for every occasion, and will be able to do away with the mad dash to try to find something to buy— something quite likely to be an expensive mistake.

Draw two pie charts. Divide the first chart into sections to reflect the amount of time you spend each day doing the following activities:

• **Working**

• **At home/looking after children**

• **Social/entertainment**

• **Leisure/hobbies**

• **Errands**

Divide the second pie chart into sections to reflect what your closet holds, using the same headings.

If you spend 50 percent of your time in the office, then 50 percent of your wardrobe should be represented by your work clothes. Likewise, if you spend only 5 percentof your time socializing, only 5 percent of your wardrobe should be for social occasions, and so on.

If the charts don't match, it's time to adjust the balance of your wardrobe so that it reflects your lifestyle.

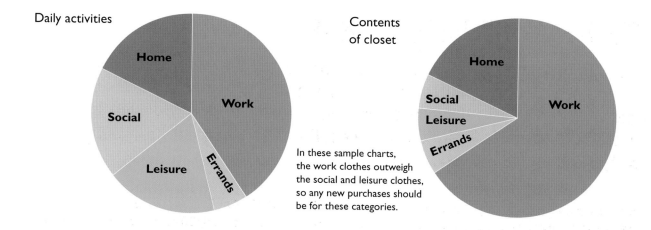

Daily activities
Home
Work
Social
Leisure
Errands

Contents of closet
Home
Social
Leisure
Work
Errands

In these sample charts, the work clothes outweigh the social and leisure clothes, so any new purchases should be for these categories.

START BY FILLING IN THE QUESTIONNAIRE BELOW

Things you like about yourself

....
....
....
....
....
....
....

Things you'd like to change

....
....
....
....
....
....

Colors

Do you wear the same colors every day?

Are there colors that you wear only at the weekend?

Are you afraid of color?

Do you tend to wear only black?

Shopping

Do you dislike shopping?

Do you have a closet full of clothes, but nothing to wear?

Do you need a different wardrobe for work?

Makeup and grooming

Have you been applying your makeup in the same way for years?

Have you had the same hairstyle for more than three years?

Whatever you have answered yes to are the issues on which you need to focus. For advice on color: go to pages 38–115. For help with your wardrobe: go to pages 116–201.

THE WELL-DRESSED WOMAN

Why is image so important? Because, as we know, in every walk of life we are judged by our appearance. When you feel good, you are automatically more confident, you stand straighter, you smile more, and you even speak with more conviction.

Has anybody ever said to you, "Are you not feeling well today?" when in fact you are feeling perfectly fine? It may simply be that you are wearing the wrong color. On the other hand, there may be occasions when you feel tired and stressed but still get complimented. At **colour me beautiful**, we're in the compliment business and we want to make sure that every day you receive compliments about the way YOU look, rather than about the clothes you are wearing.

THE KEY TO SUCCESS

Match your style personality

You will have a definite preference for a certain style of clothes, the shops you particularly like to buy from, and the way you accessorize your look. It is your style personality that will pull together the colors, lines, and shape of your clothes.

Complement your coloring

Your clothes should work in harmony and balance with the coloring of your skin, hair, and eyes. If you are dressed in the right colors, people will see more of you than the clothes you are wearing. Once you understand the right colors and styles for you, you will buy only what suits you when you go shopping. The result will be a more coordinated wardrobe.

Flatter your body lines, scale, and proportions

You will feel more comfortable wearing clothes that complement your build. An understanding of your basic shape will give you the knowledge to choose clothes that flatter your body line and balance your scale and proportions.

Choose appropriate clothes

It is important that your clothes reflect your lifestyle, whether it be professional, casual and relaxed, or formal—or a combination of all three. Not only should your clothes be appropriate for the occasion, you also need to be comfortable in the style of clothes you wear.

Look current

Nothing ages a woman more than clothes that are a decade out of fashion. Fads come and go every year, but trends stay for at least half a decade. The well-dressed woman understands the trends and may use the fads as fun items in her wardrobe.

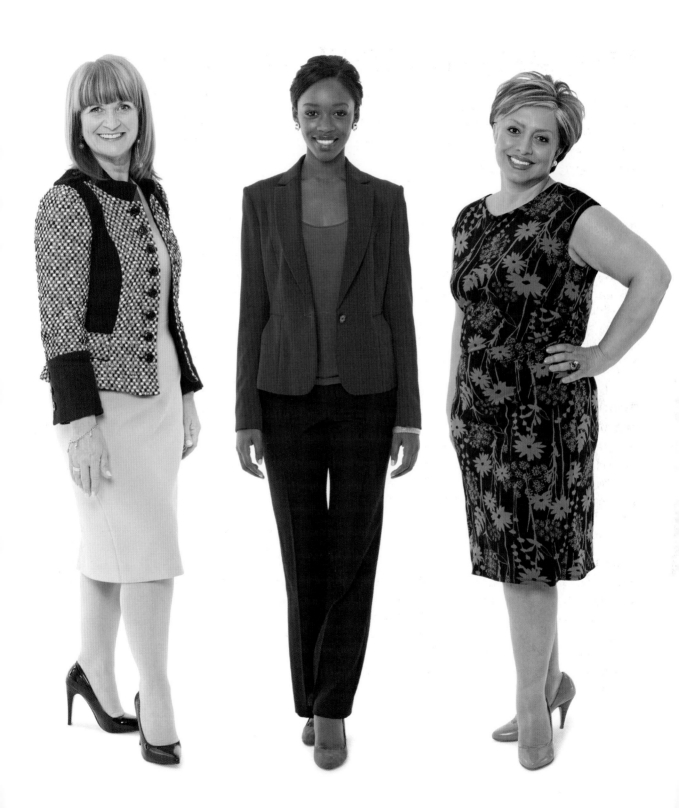

IT COULD BE YOU

Be inspired by these before and after makeovers. Each makeover is the result of a step-by-step process, and through the next few chapters you will see how it is possible to transform yourself, too.

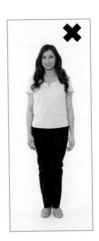

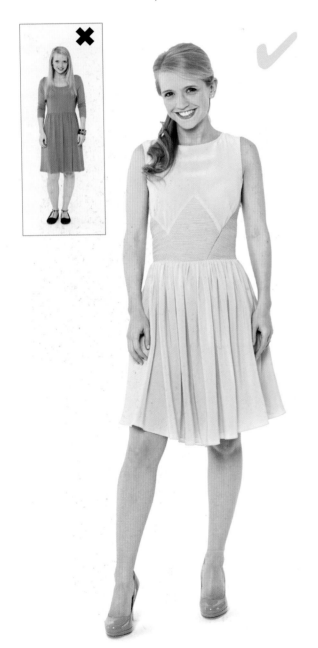

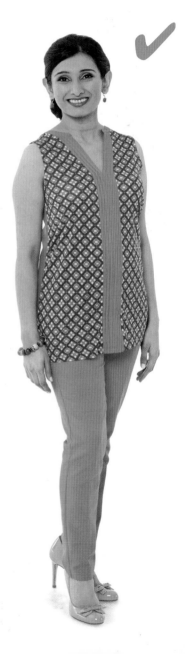

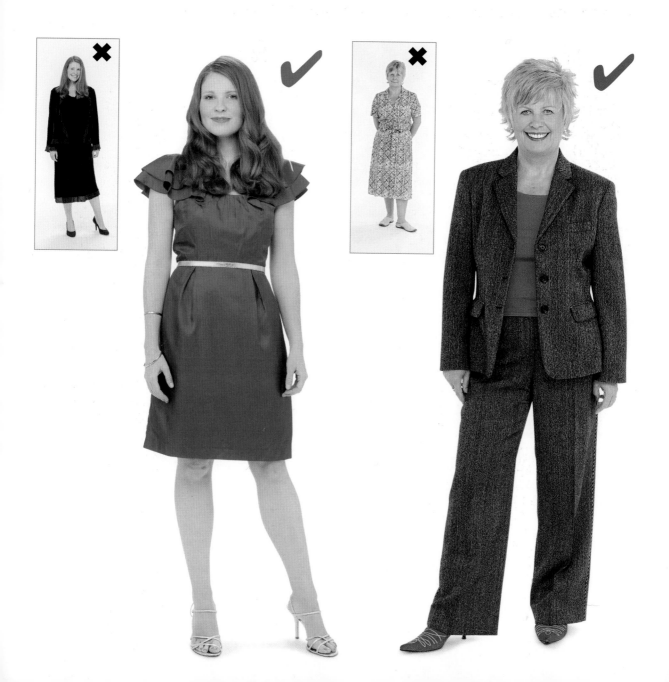

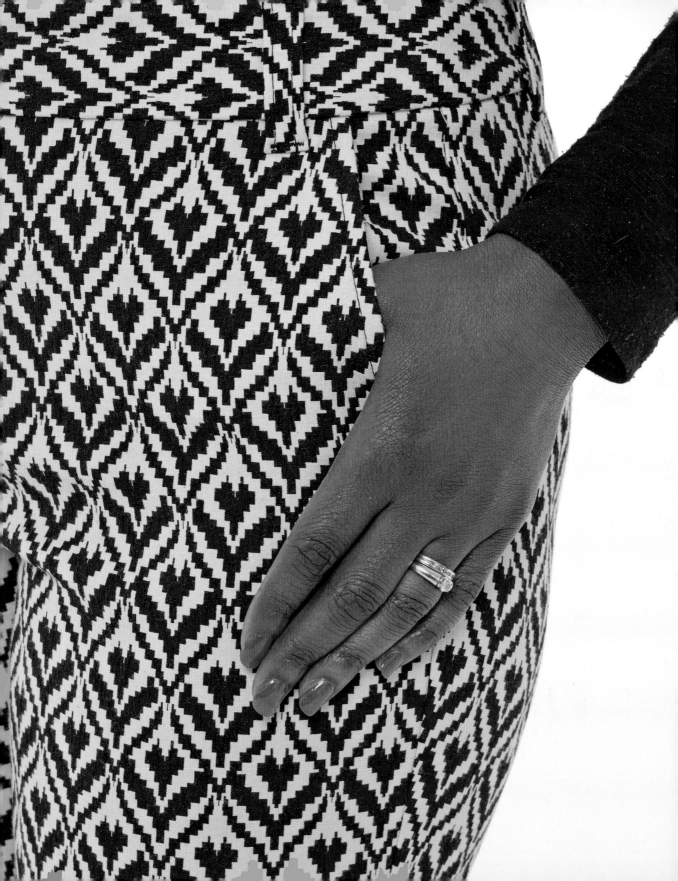

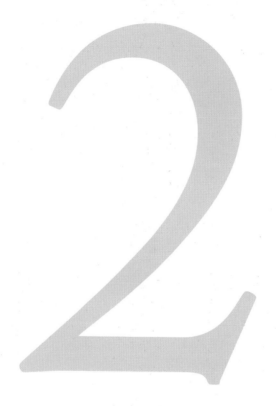

FINDING YOUR
STYLE

YOUR STYLE PERSONALITY

Naturally, the color and styling of your clothes play an important part in your appearance, but it is your personality that acts as the catalyst to pull your whole look together. Your personality dictates your style, which is your own interpretation of fashion and how you like to wear clothes.

Once you know and understand your style personality, putting your wardrobe together will become second nature. If you ignore your personality and buy clothes simply because they're featured in all the glossy magazines or look great on a friend, you will not look comfortable and your wardrobe will be a muddle of styles. This, in turn, will limit your flexibility in mixing and matching to create the perfect outfits for you. It also means that you won't get the best value from your clothing investments.

The clothes that you wear and how you wear them are governed by many factors: age, build, lifestyle, environment, budget, culture, and personal preferences. The way you project yourself may be influenced by your upbringing, the way you want others to see you, or even by a misguided approach to how you see yourself. Knowing your style personality will give you the foundation on which to project yourself in a more organized way, and to feel comfortable in your outfit, whatever the occasion.

STYLES OF THE FAMOUS

Before working out your own style personality, have a look at how famous people dress. Notice what they are wearing when they appear at their most comfortable and relaxed.

Singer Paloma Faith is a true Creative, changing her look constantly to suit her latest record or video. A trendsetter rather than a trend follower, she loves avant-garde designers.

Also a singer, Katy Perry has a Dramatic style personality, choosing clothes that get her noticed and sometimes even shock. She loves setting trends and working with the latest designers to create a look that's new and different.

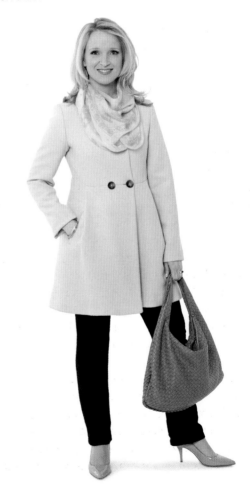

With her wonderful long, wavy hair, singer and dancer Katherine Jenkins epitomizes the Romantic style personality. On and off the red carpet, she loves pretty, feminine details and luxury fabrics.

Cristina Fernández de Kirchner, the Argentinian president, is an example of the Classic style personality. Her look is the same every time she is seen in public: simple and groomed. Nothing is out of place, nothing shocks, and she is completely coordinated.

Venus Williams, the celebrated tennis player, has a Natural style personality. She doesn't care about the world seeing her unkempt, with messy hair and without any makeup.

The Duchess of Cambridge has developed an elegance that is fashionable but not trendy. Her clothes are understated and her accessories always in vogue. It's difficult to recall exactly what she wears—you just remember that she looks good, and this is the key factor of City Chic style.

CHANGING YOUR STYLE

As you progress through life, you will feel different about the way you look. What you wear in your early twenties, for example, will be very different from how you will want to dress when middle-aged or later in life.

In your teens you might flaunt your body by wearing revealing outfits, or follow fashion fads regardless of whether they suit you. You might find yourself going out of your way to shock others through what you wear, or you may show no interest at all in clothes, personal grooming, shopping, or accessories.

As you begin to think about attracting the opposite sex, your clothes can become an extension of your sexuality. You may start to wear makeup or apply more than you used to. You may even wear really uncomfortable items of clothing simply because they help you convey how you feel inside. If you feel romantic, you may portray that emotion on the outside by wearing feminine clothes. Floral patterns may creep into your wardrobe, fabrics may become more sheer, and you may wear the odd frilly number.

As you advance in your career or become a parent, you may feel that you need a more classic look, and that you should put on a "uniform" to suit your new status in life. You start to think about making your clothes last for more than one season. Expensive investment purchases now feature in your wardrobe, and you consider how versatile an item might be before you buy it.

There are, of course, those of you who simply enjoy clothes—you're not fashion victims, but you like to look up-to-date. You have experimented over the years and have discovered what suits you, and probably have some basic items that form the core of your look. You enjoy shopping for accessories and special pieces to enhance your wardrobe. Through good advice or experimentation, you will have already learned what does and what doesn't work for you.

Some of you will have been through all these various style stages, and may feel that you are stuck in a format that's comfortable but boring. Now is the time to move on and try something new and different.

IDENTIFYING YOUR LOOK

Completing the questionnaire on the next page will help you determine your style personality. Some of you will discover that you have a split style personality, and you will need to decide which one is the most appropriate for you, although it is possible to be one type for work and another for socializing. Those of you who are really adept at planning your wardrobe might be a little of all of the personalities, depending on the occasion and how you feel at any particular time. Bear in mind that there is also a psychological aspect to color and the colors that you wear: go to pages 44–47 to explore this further.

STYLE PERSONALITY QUESTIONNAIRE

To find out your style personality, complete the questionnaire below, circling as many options as you wish. You may feel that some questions merit more than one answer—for example, one may describe how you dress during the week, another may reflect your appearance at weekends, and a third may describe how you would like to look. Take the plunge and discover the real you!

How do you wear color?

A   Whatever I feel like on the day.

B   Strong, contrasting, and bright shades.

C   Pretty pastels.

D   I like to be coordinated.

E   I do not worry about it.

F   A tone-on-tone look.

What kind of shopper are you?

A   I love markets and vintage clothes.

B   I buy something if I like it.

C   I enjoy the whole shopping experience.

D   I plan my shopping trips and take a list.

E   I shop online.

F   I am an investment buyer.

How would you describe your overall look?

A   Eclectic and sometimes wacky.

B   I like to make a statement and wear eye-catching pieces.

C   Pretty with detailed clothes that make me feel feminine.

D   Neat, organized, and coordinated.

E   Relaxed and casual.

F   Simple and elegant.

What is in your working wardrobe?

A   Interesting and different pieces.

B   Statement pieces.

C   Pretty blouses and dresses.

D   Tailored suits and coordinated pieces.

E   Easy-to-wear separates.

F   Basic pieces, but dressed up with accessories.

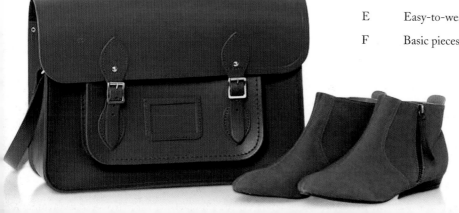

What is in your non-working wardrobe?

A   My collection of vintage clothes.

B   My latest fashion purchase.

C   Pretty, feminine pieces.

D   Coordinated separates.

E   Jeans and comfortable tops.

F   Simple styles, which I accessorize.

What is in your special occasion wardrobe?

A   Velvet, brocade, antiques, and lace.

B   Unusual and striking garments.

C   Fitted dresses with lots of detailing.

D   Simple and tailored dresses.

E   Comfortable, dressy pants or a long skirt with a loose-fitting top.

F   An elegant dress or pantsuit.

What are your shoes like?

A   They don't coordinate with my outfit.

B   High fashion styles.

C   Pretty, with bows and details.

D   They match my handbag.

E   Comfortable.

F   Current.

What kind of jewelry do you like?

A   Unusual—I collect it.

B   Bold, makes a statement.

C   Intricate, dangly, and pretty.

D   The real thing rather than fashion.

E   Minimal.

F   Current and noticeable.

What is your attitude to makeup?

A   I experiment.

B   I like it to be noticed.

C   I love it and spend time over it.

D   I keep to the same routine.

E   Minimalistic.

F   It complements my look.

What type of hairstyle do you have?

A   It changes with my mood.

B   It changes regularly.

C   Long.

D   Neat.

E   Low maintenance.

F   Up-to-date.

Once you have completed the questionnaire, count how many times you have answered A, B, and so on, and see the list on the right to determine your predominant style personality. Then refer to the following pages for examples of famous people who match your style personality and for tips on how to achieve the style successfully.

Mainly A   Creative: go to pages 26–27

Mainly B   Dramatic: go to pages 28–29

Mainly C   Romantic: go to pages 30–31

Mainly D   Classic: go to pages 32–33

Mainly E   Natural: go to pages 34–35

Mainly F   City Chic: go to pages 36–37

CREATIVE

You are great at combining different items of clothing and accessories to give yourself a unique and interesting look, and you rarely throw anything out because you know you will use it at some point, even if it has to be remodelled. If you're not careful, though, your creative tendencies could result in your being inappropriately dressed for certain occasions.

STYLE CHARACTERISTICS

- Your wardrobe is full of items from many different sources, including vintage mixed with retail and eBay purchases, which you have collected over the years.
- Shopping for you is an art form. You like nothing better than rummaging around a thrift store or your mother's attic.
- You often make interesting purchases while on vacation, and study fashion magazines for inspiration and new ideas.

MAKE THE MOST OF YOUR STYLE

- Team chunky knitwear with floaty dresses and funky boots.
- Wear pants with tunics or dresses, together with a low-slung belt.
- Make office wear a little more interesting with an eye-catching blouse or a scarf, mixed with unusual accessories.
- For the evening, choose a vintage dress, perhaps with a pair of jeweled shoes.

YOUR COLOR PALETTE

Light Primrose + light aqua; geranium + blush pink; light navy + apple green.

Deep Chocolate + eggplant; taupe + royal purple; lime + turquoise.

Warm Tangerine + mint; purple + bittersweet; charcoal + oatmeal.

Cool Light periwinkle + hot pink; duck egg + teal; blue-red + icy green.

Clear Black + apple green; light apricot + royal blue; ruby + light teal.

Soft Shell + soft violet; claret + rose brown; sage + charcoal blue.

HOW TO ACCESSORIZE

- Choose a belt that will make a statement.
- Wear a scarf that doesn't coordinate with or match what you are wearing.
- Add costume jewelry or interesting pieces as finishing touches.
- Customize clothes with interesting buttons.
- Pin a corsage or brooch to a vintage jacket to bring it up-to-date.
- Wear a hat, whatever the weather.

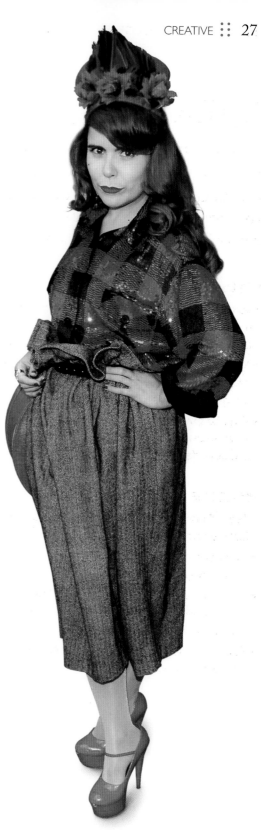

YOUR FACE

By day Choose either your eyes or your lips to create a wow effect with makeup.

By night Combine colors that do not necessarily match what you are wearing.

YOUR HAIR

Add outrageous colors to your hair. Accessorize with unusual combs, barrettes, flowers, and scarves. Experiment with braids and hair extensions.

FAMOUS CREATIVES

Paloma Faith
Beyoncé
Lady Gaga
Nicki Minaj

DRAMATIC

You always want to make an entrance. You love to be noticed and often wear clothes with a wow factor. Whatever the latest fashion, you will have to try wearing it, even if it doesn't particularly suit you. Shopping is one of your favorite pastimes. You like to party—spending a quiet evening at home reading a book is not your scene.

STYLE CHARACTERISTICS

- Your wardrobe consists of many different styles of clothes and one-off pieces that you have bought on impulse, without a thought as to whether you have anything to wear with them.
- Your friends are often envious of your striking appearance and style.
- You are not concerned with whether your clothes are practical or washable—they must simply make a statement.
- You will scour the fashion press for the latest trends and ideas.

MAKE THE MOST OF YOUR STYLE

- Wear separates in contrasting colors.
- The bolder and more striking your accessories, the better.
- In the evening, wear that "Oscar" dress; it's your style to dress up, rather than down, for parties and special occasions.
- Be prepared to tone down your look for daytime in the office.

YOUR COLOR PALETTE

Light Light gray + geranium; peacock + blush pink; taupe + violet.

Deep Black + soft white; scarlet + damson plum; chocolate + fern.

Warm Purple + amber; bronze + daffodil; orange-red + aqua.

Cool Charcoal + periwinkle; cassis + royal blue; spruce + blue-green.

Clear True blue + ivory; apple green + light apricot; true red + black-brown.

Soft Purple + light periwinkle; emerald turquoise + mint; rose brown + claret.

HOW TO ACCESSORIZE

- Wear belts with interesting buckles and details, such as studs, jewels, or cut-out patterns.
- Make a statement by choosing bold patterns in contrasting colors.
- Wear large, striking jewelry, but don't wear too much at once.
- Update your look each season with new shoes or boots.
- Throw a colorful scarf over your winter coat.
- Make your handbag a statement one.

YOUR FACE

By day Don't forget your eye pencil plus two or three coats of mascara, and your lip gloss.

By night Nothing but the full works for you, finished off with a red lipstick.

YOUR HAIR

Add a striking color to your hair (in tones that complement your coloring). Change your hairstyle regularly and consult your hairdresser to ensure you keep up with the latest styles. Use hair treatments and styling products to keep your hair in peak condition at all times.

FAMOUS DRAMATICS

Katy Perry
Christina Hendricks
Chaka Khan
Serena Williams

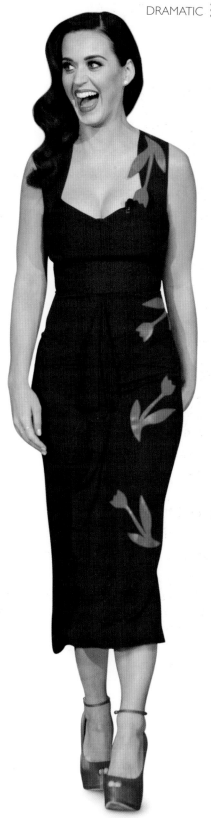

ROMANTIC

You love everything about dressing up and planning your wardrobe. Your clothes are pretty and you adore all sorts of details: bows, ruffles, flounces, appliqués, and fringes. You love to experiment with new skincare and bodycare products, and never go out without your perfume. You will spend longer than anybody else looking after yourself and your grooming.

STYLE CHARACTERISTICS

- Flowers feature heavily in your wardrobe, whether they are in patterned fabrics or as accessories and decorative details, such as corsages, brooches, and other jewelry.
- You always wear matching and pretty underwear, even if it is uncomfortable.
- Your sports clothes are either in pretty colors or have decorative details.
- Even your everyday work clothes are pretty, feminine, and detailed.

MAKE THE MOST OF YOUR STYLE

- Choose separates that are decorated with beading, appliqué, or ribbons.
- Choose luxury fabrics such as angora, cashmere, silk, and satin.
- Skirts or dresses teamed with a cardigan or pretty jacket are a great look for you.
- In the evening, go for a layered look and choose fabrics such as chiffon or lace decorated with sequins and diamanté. Complete the look by wearing high-heeled sandals.

YOUR COLOR PALETTE

Light Light navy + pastel pink; pewter + mint; light aqua + light apricot.

Deep Charcoal + blush pink; cornflower + primrose; eggplant + olive.

Warm Coral + cream; gray-green + teal; amber + taupe.

Cool Rose pink + baby pink; sky blue + medium gray; bright periwinkle + icy green.

Clear Emerald turquoise + duck egg; scarlet + light gray; royal blue + light apricot.

Soft Blush pink + soft violet; spruce + mint; cocoa + shell.

HOW TO ACCESSORIZE

- Add a flower somewhere: in your hair, on your shoulder, to your bag, or even your shoes.
- Floral prints work well if you have soft, curvier body lines; if you don't, choose spots or squiggles.
- Wear decorative jewelry.
- Colorful, pretty handbags are perfect for you.
- Wear fine-patterned or textured tights; seamed stockings are fun if you have shapely legs and ankles.
- Always wear a heel, whether on a sandal or boot.

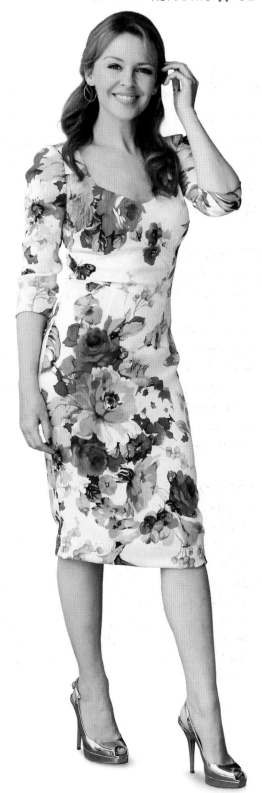

YOUR FACE

By day You always wear makeup, especially a pink lipstick and a blusher from your palette.

By night For an ultra-feminine look, dazzle with sparkle, shimmer, and glitter.

YOUR HAIR

The best hairstyles for you are long and layered, softly curled and probably highlighted. Put decorations in your hair if you wear it up.

FAMOUS ROMANTICS

Kylie Minogue
Penélope Cruz
Leona Lewis
Aung San Suu Kyi

CLASSIC

You have a fairly formal wardrobe. You like to appear well dressed and elegant, and your tops are usually tucked in. You are content to keep to the same hairstyles, and hate it when your hairdresser moves away. Your makeup routine is fixed and you rarely experiment with new shades. You have a few favorite stores that you visit when you need new clothes.

STYLE CHARACTERISTICS

- Your look is timeless and neat.
- You prefer a coordinated look and do not like to mix textures or wear daring color combinations.
- Your workwear is smart and understated.
- At weekends you are likely to replace your jacket and blouse with coordinated separates.
- You rarely wear jeans, preferring a pair of classic pants teamed with leather loafers.
- You do not follow fashion.

MAKE THE MOST OF YOUR STYLE

- Coordinated separates are the basis of all your looks.
- By mixing and matching what you already have you will create many more outfits.
- Add colored tops to your basic jackets to achieve a more varied look.
- Your evening wear will be simple, to which you will add your favorite pieces of jewelry.

YOUR COLOR PALETTE

Light Stone + cornflower; light navy + dusty rose; cocoa + light aqua.

Deep Charcoal + burgundy; black-brown + olive; pewter + teal.

Warm Gray-green + oatmeal; chocolate + cream; bronze + amber.

Cool Dark navy + icy blue; pine + light teal; medium gray + rose pink.

Clear Black + duck egg; dark navy + emerald turquoise; taupe + blush pink.

Soft Natural beige + verbena; charcoal blue + shell; chocolate + mint.

HOW TO ACCESSORIZE

- Match your handbag and shoes.
- Add quality costume jewelry to the real thing to create a more varied look.
- The quickest way for you to update your look is with a new pair of shoes in the latest style.
- Change your handbag regularly.
- Do not wear all your favorite pieces of matching jewelry at the same time.
- A scarf will always finish your look.

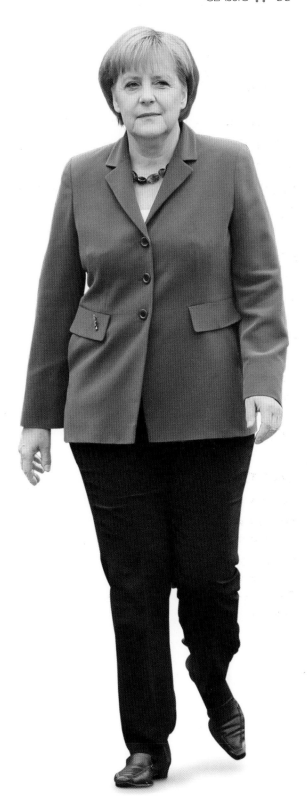

YOUR FACE

By day Don't be afraid to try some new eye shadow and lipstick colors once in a while.

By night Go one or two tones darker within your coloring.

YOUR HAIR

Consider changing your hairstyle every two or three years, keeping your color as close to your natural shade as possible. Your preferred styles are easy to manage without complicated styling techniques.

FAMOUS CLASSICS

Angela Merkel
Hillary Clinton
Princess Anne
Cristina Fernández de Kirchner

NATURAL

Feeling comfortable in your clothes is the most important factor for you when choosing what to wear; anything that constricts, digs in, or pinches is not an option. You prefer casual styling to formal business wear, and you hate a cluttered look—simple lines and designs are more you. In keeping with your no-fuss attitude, clothes must be easy-care and ideally non-iron.

STYLE CHARACTERISTICS

• Your closet may appear disorganized and you will often just wear whatever is at hand and clean that morning.

• Pants worn with flat shoes are your preferred option for maximum comfort and practicality.

• You have many interests, but reading fashion magazines is not one of them.

• Your jewelry will be minimal—if you wear any at all—and won't jangle about.

MAKE THE MOST OF YOUR STYLE

• Long skirts—either full, pleated, or with a split—will allow freedom of movement; team them with boots or comfortable shoes.

• Go for deconstructed and loose-fitting clothes for a relaxed look.

• For work, comfort is still important, so opt for a simple, good-quality top.

• For evening, try a tunic-type top over a pair of silk pants with flat pumps.

YOUR COLOR PALETTE

Light Stone + cornflower; medium gray + dusty rose; light navy + light aqua.

Deep Black + eggplant; dark navy + purple; stone + true red.

Warm Dark brown + terracotta; moss + cream; teal + turquoise.

Cool Rose beige + sapphire; pewter + bright periwinkle; pine + light gray.

Clear Black + evergreen; purple + lemon yellow; taupe + Chinese blue.

Soft Stone + claret; cocoa + jade; damson plum + shell.

HOW TO ACCESSORIZE

• Your accessories will be minimal, but you still need them to complete your look.

• Wear a long scarf or pashmina over your coat or jacket, teamed with a pair of colorful gloves.

• For jewelry, choose natural materials such as wood, leather, and shell.

• A backpack-style handbag or one with a long shoulder strap is best for you.

• Keep your shoes comfortable but well maintained.

YOUR FACE

By day Your makeup is minimal, so all-in-one products like tinted moisturizer are ideal.

By night You don't tend to change your makeup dramatically for the evening; simply add a fresh slick of a natural-colored lipstick or gloss.

YOUR HAIR

You don't like to spend much time on your tresses, so it's essential to have a good haircut that allows you to leave your hair to dry with little or no styling.

FAMOUS NATURALS

Emily Blunt
Julia Roberts
Venus Williams
Kate Winslet

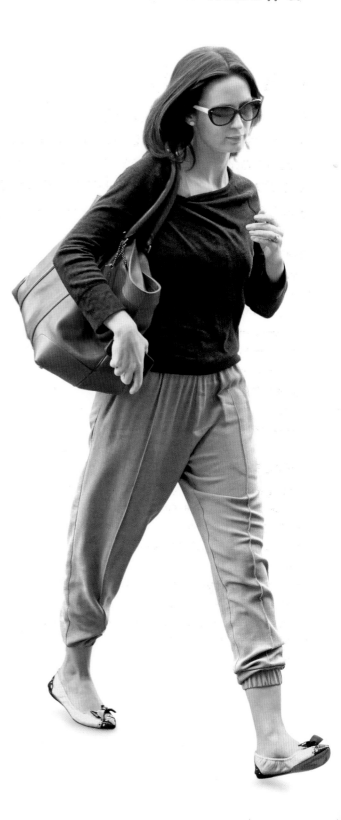

CITY CHIC

You enjoy your clothes but are not fanatical about them. You dedicate time and thought to the way you look, and you love accessories, sometimes spending more on bags and shoes than on an outfit itself. Having probably tried out most of the other key styles and experimented with lots of different looks, you now know what suits you.

STYLE CHARACTERISTICS

- You tend to follow trends rather than retail fashion.
- You shop with care and rarely make rash purchases, ensuring that whatever you buy coordinates with other items that you already have in your wardrobe.
- You use bright colors with caution and tend to go for a tone-on-tone look.
- You keep abreast of the latest trends by reading women's magazines.

MAKE THE MOST OF YOUR STYLE

- Invest in basic, classic pieces in neutral colors.
- Keep your working wardrobe updated with new tops, purchased regularly.
- Team pants with a stylish shirt or twin-set and accessorize appropriately.
- For evening, a simple shift dress with a stunning necklace, worn with a colorful wrap or pashmina, will be a great success. Pumps would be a good choice for footwear to complete this simple but stylish outfit.

YOUR COLOR PALETTE

Light Stone + cocoa; light periwinkle + sky blue; pastel pink + dusty rose.

Deep Black + charcoal; pine + mint; purple + damson plum.

Warm Bronze + moss; bittersweet + terracotta; daffodil + amber.

Cool Medium gray + light gray; light periwinkle + dark periwinkle; cassis + rose pink.

Clear True blue + royal blue; evergreen + emerald green; pewter + light teal.

Soft Cocoa + rose brown; sage + spruce; damson plum + soft violet.

HOW TO ACCESSORIZE

- Make a statement with a single accessory, be it a stunning necklace, brooch, or beaded scarf.
- Even when it's not sunny, always wear your sunglasses somewhere, such as on your head.
- Swap the black handbag for a colorful one.
- Tie a scarf to your handbag.
- Wear a quality watch.
- Wear an elegant heeled pump shoe with your pants.

YOUR FACE

By day Create a matte finish for your face, and add a touch of bronzer and a neutral lipstick.

By night Enhance your eye makeup with a granite or brown pencil and add a little sheen or gloss to your eyelids; enhance your lips with a darker shade.

YOUR HAIR

Keep your hair in good condition and have it cut regularly. Subtle highlights and lowlights will ensure a natural look.

FAMOUS CITY CHICS

Halle Berry
Duchess of Cambridge
Christine Lagarde
Freida Pinto

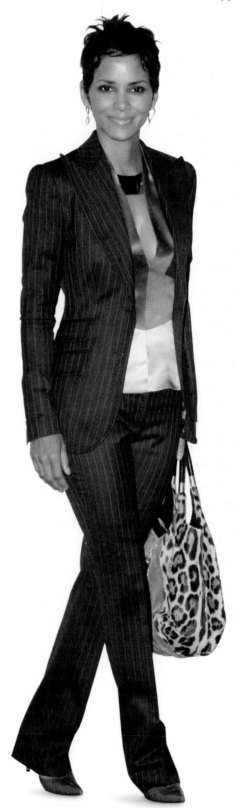

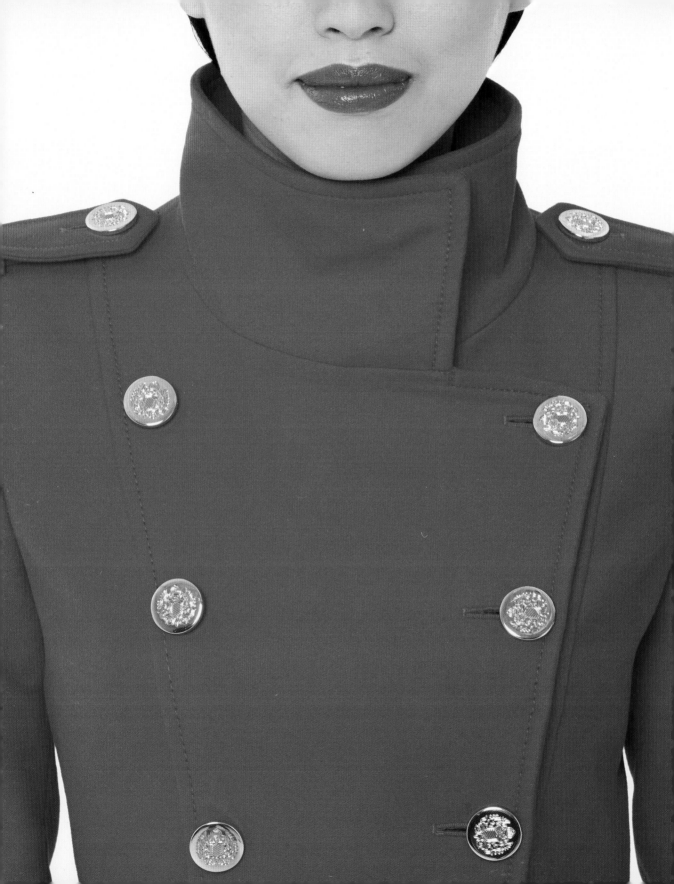

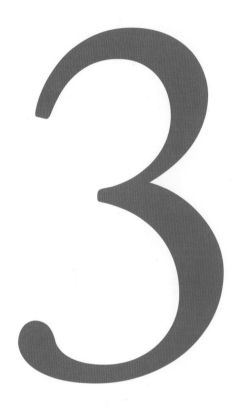

UNDERSTANDING COLOR

FINDING YOUR COLORS

Color can be magical. Seeing a flash of color emerge from a largely monochromatic crowd is energizing, like a breath of fresh air; and once you start wearing colors, there will be no stopping you. For many years neutral colors held sway in fashion, but now that color—in all its hues— is back, the time is right to learn how to make colors work for you. So let us take you on a colorful and stylish journey.

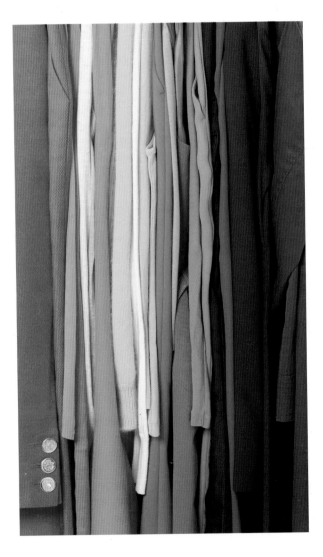

IF YOU KNOW YOUR COLORING

• Shopping will become easier, the choice of colors second nature.

• You will always have in your wardrobe the right combination of colors to wear.

• You will gain confidence from knowing that the colors you are wearing are those that flatter.

• You will be on the exciting path to a new you.

HOW COLOR WORKS

When you wear color near your face, the light reflects it upward; this can cast either flattering tones or dark shadows, depending on the mix of the color and your skin tone. This is one reason why it is important to work out your dominant coloring type and discover which are the right colors for you: go to pages 48–49.

There is a psychological aspect to color, too, and the colors you wear can communicate non-verbal messages of various kinds. Soft and light tones, for example, will make you appear approachable and friendly, while a red top in the right shade will help to give you the confidence you need when facing a stressful situation. Colors that you might wear on a first date with a man you wish to impress will probably not be suitable at a school parents' evening, nor at an important business meeting where you want to appear in control: go to pages 44–47.

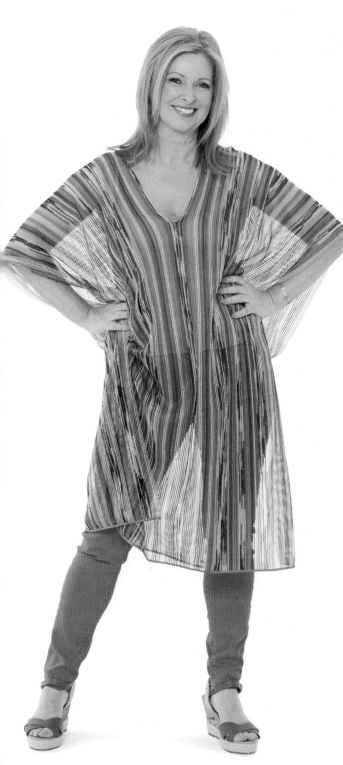

THE TIME OF YOUR LIFE

We are all born with perfect skin, beautiful eyes, and healthy hair, the colors of which are all genetically balanced together. Over the years environment, diet, and everyday stresses can all take their toll on how we look. You may, for example, live in a climate where your natural hair color becomes sun-streaked and your skin acquires a tan.

When the hormones start up—first in your teens and then again at the time of menopause—it's all change again. If you look at a photograph of yourself as a young child, and then as a teenager, you may well see a marked difference in hair color. The gorgeous platinum blonde child has now become a young woman with dark blonde hair. That young girl who had the most wonderful jet-black hair starts to see natural highlights appear, especially white or gray hair at her parting or temples, and the very bright colors she used to wear may now start to overpower her. It is always more difficult for those with darker hair tones to hide these signs of aging in a flattering way and sometimes it is best to let nature take its course or even look at changing your dominant coloring type. Dark brown hair with gray showing can look stunning when warm tones are added, taking someone from Deep to Warm.

If you were color analyzed some years ago, you may now have changed and feel less happy wearing certain recommended colors. For this reason, the idea that a person is one "season" or palette all their life is no longer true. So, if you have been following a "seasonal" palette for some time, it may now be time to review your coloring.

THE SCIENCE OF COLOR

There are two main influences behind **colour me beautiful**'s current approach to color—those of Johannes Itten and Alfred Munsell. The seasonal color concept that lay behind the original **colour me beautiful**—and which lasted for more than 20 years—was first developed in the 1920s by the artist Johannes Itten of the Bauhaus school. Itten noticed that his students always did their best work using colors they had chosen themselves. In his book, *The Art of Color*, Itten reveals the strong relationship between a student's appearance, their personality, and the colors they liked to work with.

This concept was further developed at the Fashion Academy of Los Angeles, founded in 1972. Former student Carole Jackson made the seasonal concept popular in her book, *Color Me Beautiful*, published in 1980. The book was translated into many languages and for months remained on the *New York Times* bestseller list. In 1986 Doris Pooser developed Carole Jackson's seasonal concept further, but with the addition of the Munsell theory (see opposite), in her book, *Always in Style*.

Over the past 30 years, **colour me beautiful** has moved from a seasonal color analysis system to the methods that we use today, which are based on the Munsell system. With fashion constantly on the move, it is impossible to give accurate samples of colors to our clients. Fabric, texture, and weaves also have an effect on how the human eye sees color. We now like to educate our clients in *how* to wear color rather than *what* color to wear. The beauty of Munsell's system is that it can be used to describe a person's coloring as well as to specify the colors they should wear, the aim always being to create harmony and balance between the two. The theory behind his system is that all colors have one dominant characteristic and one or two secondary characteristics. A person's coloring will also have one dominant characteristic. For the purpose of this book we will be only dealing with the dominant characteristic, giving a reliable, versatile, and easy-to-follow way of using colors for all.

THE MUNSELL SYSTEM

Munsell's is the most widely accepted system of color measurement; it is used by both the U.S. National Bureau of Standards and the British Standards Institution. So, who was Munsell? In 1903 Albert Munsell—also an artist—invented a system of color identification based on the responses of the human eye. In 1905 his *System of Color Notation* became

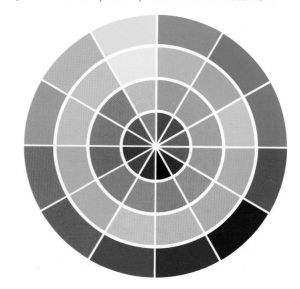

universally recognized as the language of color. In this, colors were identified as having three characteristics: hue, value, and chroma.

The uses of this "language" are innumerable, particularly in the building, printing, and motor industries. The Munsell system is even used to codify all tints and dyes within the hairdressing industry. So if you color your hair, you are already using the Munsell system.

All three Munsell characteristics—hue, value, and chroma—can be referred to when describing a color.

HUE–UNDERTONE

Hue defines a color's undertone, which may be warm (yellow-based) or cool (blue-based). Colors such as red, pink, and green can be described as having either a warm or a cool undertone. You might have a cool "blue" red (say, a plum-colored red) or a warm "orange" red (a tomato red); likewise, you can have a warm olive green (yellow-based) or a cool pine green (blue-based).

VALUE–DEPTH

The value of a color refers to its depth, giving a measure of its lightness or darkness. Munsell used a scale of 0 to 10, with black being 0 and white being 10, and with all the shades of gray in between. This grading of light and dark can be used to measure the depth of all other colors, too; for example, in hairdressing these numbers determine the depth of color of a hair dye.

CHROMA–CLARITY

Chroma indicates the purity or clarity of a color. Some colors are bright and vibrant and reflect the light, while others are dusty or muted and seem to absorb light. The type of fabric in question will also determine whether light is absorbed or reflected; for example, satin reflects light, while wool seems to absorb it. The chroma scale ranges from 0 to 14, with 0 being the most grayed or muted and 14 being the clearest.

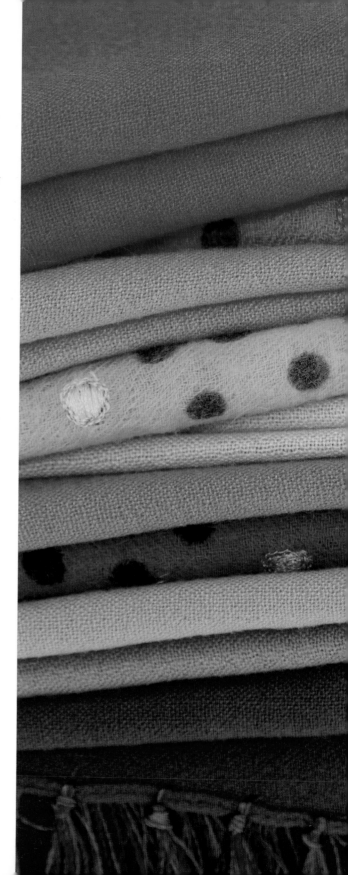

THE PSYCHOLOGY OF COLOR

Much research has been done on the psychology of color and its effects on everyday life. Color can affect your mood and your energy levels profoundly, and therefore has a great impact on your general sense of wellbeing. It will also affect how others view you, from your partner to your boss.

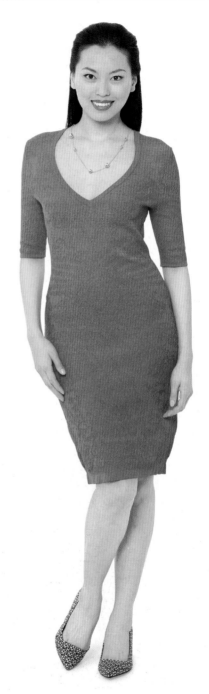

Before you get to find out about your own coloring type, let us first take a look at the psychological effect on yourself and others when you wear certain colors. This is not only gleaned from the extensive results of scientific research but also from the knowledge and vast experience that **colour me beautiful** has gained over the years in the course of meeting so many women.

COLOR AND WHAT IT MEANS

Being able to distinguish between varying hues and strengths of color makes it plausible to assume that colors impact our behavior, just as our senses of taste, smell, touch, and hearing cause us to respond to external signals. Over recent years much research has been carried out by eminent scientists to find out why sports teams wearing red win more often—countries whose Olympic teams' strips are red continually win more medals. Red is a color that is seen as assertive and sometimes aggressive. Similarly, it has been known for many years that blue and green have a calming effect, and that yellow makes us feel happy. Making the right choice of color to suit the occasion is just as important as choosing one that works for us. Note, too, that colors have certain relevance in different cultures.

BLACK/GRAY

Black can portray an air of authority and it is worn by many women as a uniform for business

Wearing black from head to toe every day is easy and safe, but may give the message that you lack imagination. It also implies that you are hiding behind the color. It might be a good idea to wear black with another color for greater impact. For example, a little black evening dress can be a winner; if black is not in your palette, wear it with accessories near your face (pearls or beads) that tone well with your natural coloring. A pashmina or chiffon scarf in your colors will be perfect. Or, you could wear a suitable gray—either charcoal, medium gray, or pewter—instead.

BROWN

Brown, the color of the earth, is a great color to wear when you're in relaxed mode

The brown family comes in many guises: chocolate, coffee, mahogany, and golden, to name but a few. Brown denotes a friendly, down-to-earth, though serious, attitude. We are often told that brown is "this season's black," and it provides an excellent alternative for those with Warm coloring, especially when you want to appear less threatening. Brown may be considered boring when worn on its own, but mixing it with other colors can bring it to life and it could become a staple of your casual and work wardrobe. Make sure you choose the correct shade for you by checking which tone of brown is in your dominant palette.

BEIGE

This family of colors is a great substitute for black and browns in summer

The beiges run from stone to camel via taupe, pewter, cocoa, and natural. All of these tones are non-threatening, friendly, and approachable; they are excellent when you want people to open up to you. They are ideal colors for anyone who works with people, for example in counseling, human resources, and nursing. If your coloring is either Deep (pages 62–71) or Clear (pages 92–101), beige generally needs to be worn together with contrasting deeper shades. The joy of these tones is that they may be worn all year round with the fashion colors from your palette.

WHITE

White denotes purity and freshness

Everyone needs white in their palette, whether worn head to toe for a special outing or as a contrast against other colors from your palette. It can be a hard color to wear in its purest form, but there are shades of white to suit everyone, from soft white to ivory and cream; once you have identified your dominant coloring type on the following pages, refer to your color palette to see which shade is the best for you. Wearing white in a textured fabric will often soften its appearance. Linen and silk, for example, are rarely a pure white, although cotton can be. White is an ideal color to wear in hot climates, as it reflects light—the challenge is keeping it clean and fresh-looking.

BLUE

Blue, the color of logic, activates the mind

Blue conveys trust, peace, and order—it could be considered "safe." When a leading British scarf retailer commissioned a survey to find out which colors sold best, blue came in first. Dark navy is often associated with authority and law and order; many police forces use navy for their uniforms. Medium shades of blue, such as cornflower, lapis, and sapphire, are all great colors to brighten up your wardrobe throughout the year. The lighter shades, such as powder blue, eau de nil, bluebell, and sky blue, make wonderful colors for special occasions when a feminine look may be required. Teamed with darker shades (navy and gray), they become great colors for shirts and tops.

PINK

Wearing pink suggests gentleness and empathy; it brings out the femininity in every woman

All women need some pink in their wardrobe, whether it is for a robe, some underwear, or a pashmina. Wearing a pale pink outfit will not be a powerful statement, but a blush pink or rose pink worn under a business suit will soften your look. Or, wow them on the dance floor with any shade of pink from apricot to fuchsia—but not worn head to toe in the daytime. Pink is a great color to wear when you are feeling a little off color, as it gives a flattering lift to any complexion.

PURPLE

In its pure form, purple shows creativity as well as indicating sensitivity

The purple family runs from softest lavender to deepest damson plum. It is a great alternative—and a more exciting one—to black and navy. Beware that its creative signal does not compromise a situation where you want to appear conformist. Purple is also the color of spiritualism and meditation. In its lighter forms, the lilacs and soft violets promote a general sense of relaxation. Many people shy away from purple, but if you've never worn it, give it a try in a scarf or pashmina. You'll be amazed at the effect it has on others.

RED

Red is the color of energy; wear red and you will feel confident and in control

The red family has many variations, from raspberry to tomato, so getting the undertone right is crucial. Is it warm (yellow-based) or cool (blue-based)? Wearing red will bring excitement into your day. It is the color of stimulation, showing a sense of exhilaration but also suggesting a demanding character. It is a great color to wear at the end of the week when your energy levels may be flagging. Do not, however, wear red when trying to calm children at bedtime. When wearing red, take care over choosing your lipstick. Make sure it is in the same tone, although it can be lighter or darker.

GREEN

Green, the color of grass and leaves, conveys a sense of calm and reassurance

When wearing green, whether olive or lime, or anything in between, you show creativity and imagination. It was once thought to be unlucky, but in the world of fashion, green brings another dimension to the wardrobe. With all its various shades, green may be used for virtually any garment, from a winter coat to a fun pair of shoes. With green, it is particularly important to understand the undertone and to know whether you are better in a warm (yellow-based) green, such as moss or apple green, or the cool (blue-based) green of spruce or sea green.

GAINING COLOR CONFIDENCE

All you need to do to work out which are the best colors for you is to follow the simple steps outlined below. Each coloring type is covered in more detail in Chapter 4, Your Color Type, on pages 50–115.

STEP 1 – FIND YOUR DOMINANT COLORING

- Do you have light hair and light eyes? Go to page 52.
- Do you have dark hair and dark eyes and maybe dark skin? Go to page 62.
- Does your hair have red tones? Go to page 72.
- Do you have gray or completely black hair? Go to page 82.
- Is your hair dark, but you have bright or light eyes? Go to page 92.
- Or are you a mixture of all and don't fit anywhere else? Go to page 102.

Read through the section that applies to you to understand which neutrals and fashion colors will work for you.

...AND IDENTIFY YOUR DOMINANT COLORING TYPE

In each dominant section we have three different coloring types. The variations may relate to skin tone, eye color, or the depth of hair color. Look more closely at the celebrity examples as well as at the models on the recommended pages and see which one you feel you look most like. Warm skin tones will have a yellow or golden undertone while cool skins are often pinkish in color or blue toned. Some people have neither a warm or cool skin undertone to their skin—they have a neutral skin. The undertone of your skin will not be affected if your skin tans in the sun.

STEP 2 – THE COLOR TEST

Find examples of the suggested colors, using scarves, tops or any other garment that you can easily hold near your face. If necessary, borrow from your friends.

Sit in front of a mirror with no makeup on. Make sure you are in a well-lit area, with no shadows falling on your face. Natural daylight is preferable. Hold each of the suggested colors in turn under your chin and look at the result. Does the color show on your chin? Does the color make your complexion change?

You'll know the color is right when:

- Your face appears to be lit from underneath.
- Your skin appears smoother, fresher, and younger; lines and blemishes are minimized.
- Your eye color is enhanced.
- You notice YOU more than the color.

You'll identify the wrong colors when:

- There are dark or colored shadows around your chin and neck.
- Your complexion looks uneven in color.
- The color stands out more than you.

STEP 3 – CONFIRM YOUR COLOR TYPE
Am I a Light?

Lights only look good in light colors. See how you feel when you wear your favorite light color near your face. Do you feel radiant and happy? Now try black, then charcoal and then medium gray. If the medium gray is best then you are Light.

Am I a Deep?

Deeps look good in really dark strong colors. Try yourself, in black. Do you feel confident and happy in it? Now try a pale color near your face; does it make you look pale? Do you feel you need to add a stronger lipstick? If the dark colors work best then you are probably Deep.

Am I a Warm?

Warms only look good in warm shades, that is a color with a yellow/warm undertone such as a salmon pink, or moss green rather than a fuchsia pink or pine green which have a blue/cool undertone. See how you feel when you try salmon pink compared with fuchsia pink. If you are Warm you will look better in the salmon and moss.

Am I a Cool?

Cools only look good in cool shades—that is a color with a blue/cool undertone such as fuchsia pink or pine green rather than yellow/warm tones such as salmon pink or moss. See how you feel when you try fuchsia pink compared with salmon pink. If you are Cool the fuchsia pink and pine green will be best.

Am I a Clear?

Clears look good in really bright jewel-like colors such as emerald green and clear red. Try and compare yourself in these colors against tones of soft jade or rust. If the bright colors are best then you are Clear.

Am I a Soft?

Softs look good in a blended tonal look and often are not happy wearing bright red. A great way to see if you are Soft is to compare a soft jade green with a bright emerald green; if the jade looks best then you are Soft.

For someone who is Light, the color test will reveal that a pale pink is more flattering than a deep fuchsia.

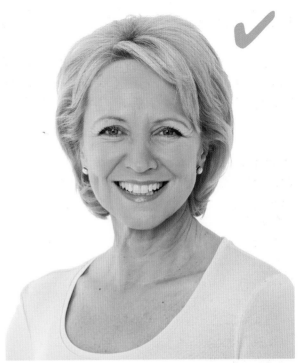

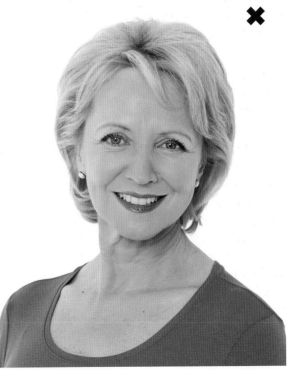

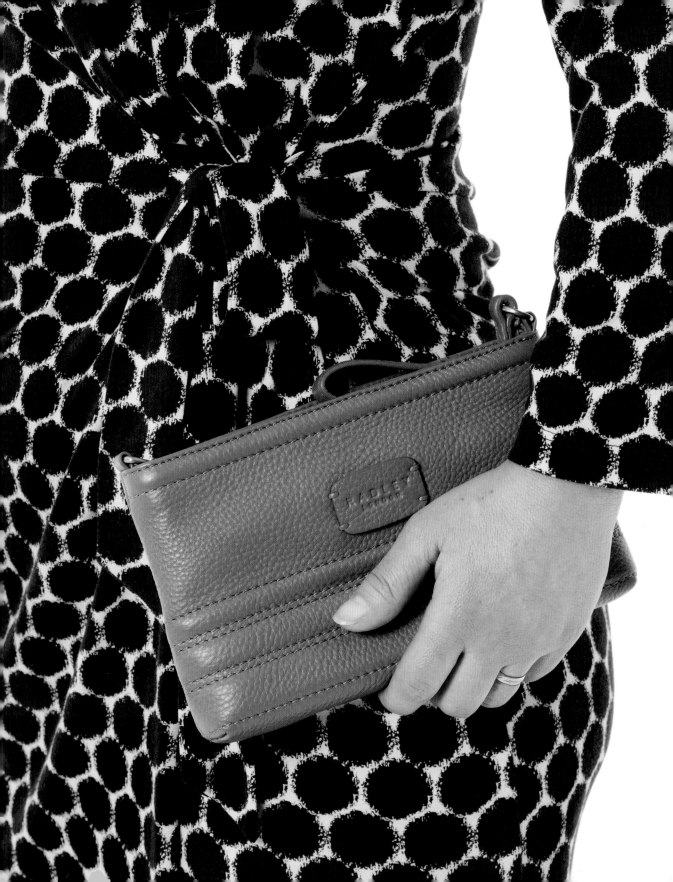

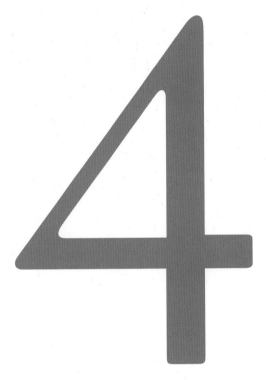

YOUR COLOR TYPE

ARE YOU A LIGHT ?

DO YOU HAVE . . .

- Naturally blonde or very light hair?
- Pale blue, gray, or light green eyes?
- Pale eyelashes?
- Pale or indistinguishable eyebrows that you often pencil in?
- Delicate skin, probably porcelain in tone, that burns easily in the sun?

YOUR LOOK IS

- Light and delicate.
- The undertone of your skin may be warm or cool.
- The depth of your coloring is light.
- The clarity of your look may be either clear or soft.

YOUR IDEAL COLORS

For a master color palette: go to pages 54–55.

HOW TO WEAR YOUR COLORS

Balance your dominant look by wearing light or medium-depth color near your face. If you have to choose a darker tone, such as light navy, for a jacket, try to contrast it with a light shade such as light apricot, rather than with a deep one like geranium.

Wear two light colors together or a combination of light and dark—but never wear two dark colors together. Always have the lighter colors close to your face.

BE AWARE

Shopping may be a challenge in the winter season, especially when you are looking for a coat or jacket,

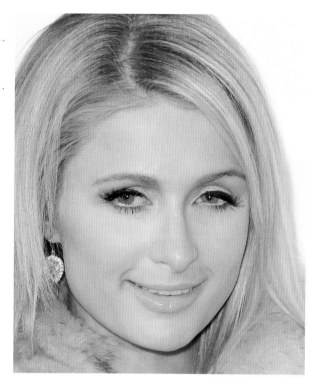

Paris Hilton is the lightest of all our Lights with her light blonde hair, pale eyebrows, and light blue eyes.

as these are traditionally dark in color. You can try rose brown—or wear a scarf or pashmina in a light shade over your coat.

BEING A LIGHT THROUGH THE AGES

If you are Light when you reach your twenties you will remain a Light throughout your life, unless you decide to dramatically change your hair coloring. Your features (eyebrows and eyelashes) will remain pale throughout your life.

Some women will become Light as they mature as their whole coloring fades; their hair actually goes white and they lose definition in their eye color as well. This often happens when they reach their late sixties

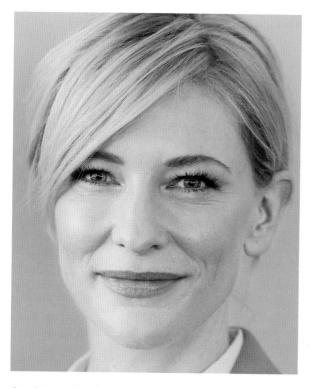

Cate Blanchett has slightly more definition to her look but is still a natural blonde, with blue eyes and porcelain skin.

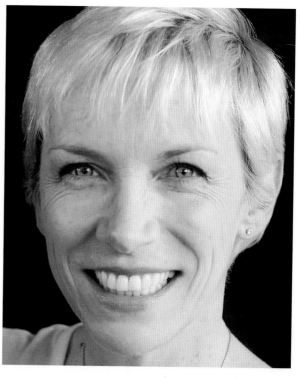

Annie Lennox is someone whose coloring has lightened over the years, and looks wonderful with her pale ash blonde hair.

or even later. Strong colors from other palettes will overpower them but the soft and pale colors of the light palette will flatter them.

WEARING YOUR PALETTE

- Use your deepest colors for your investment buys, such as your jackets, skirts, and pants. Then add the fashion colors near your face to balance your look.

- Light colors will always draw attention to where they are worn so if you are full busted, for example, one of your darker shades worn on the top half will be more flattering.

- For workwear, see the colors for the capsule wardrobe on page 171.

COLORING YOUR HAIR

Lightest blonde   Light blonde   Pale ash blonde

A Light's hair color will always be a natural blonde whether ash or strawberry; her hair could be mixed with white too. If the color fades, always go lighter rather than darker.

LIGHT COLOR PALETTE

INVESTMENT COLORS

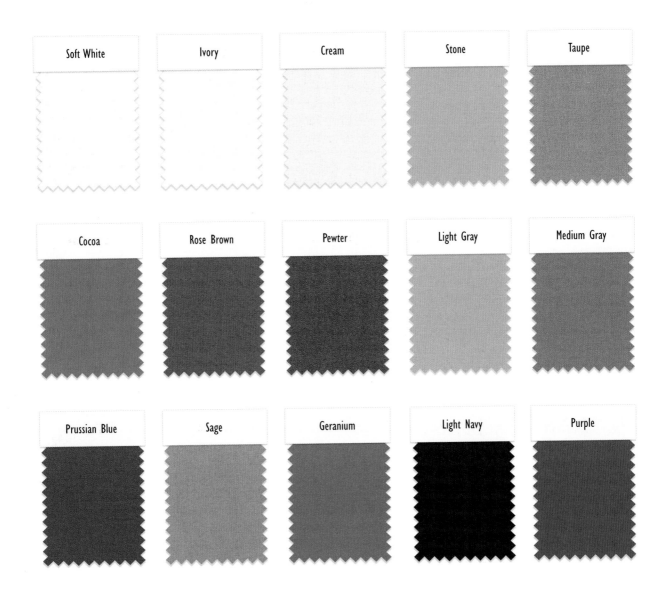

Soft White   Ivory   Cream   Stone   Taupe

Cocoa   Rose Brown   Pewter   Light Gray   Medium Gray

Prussian Blue   Sage   Geranium   Light Navy   Purple

FASHION COLORS

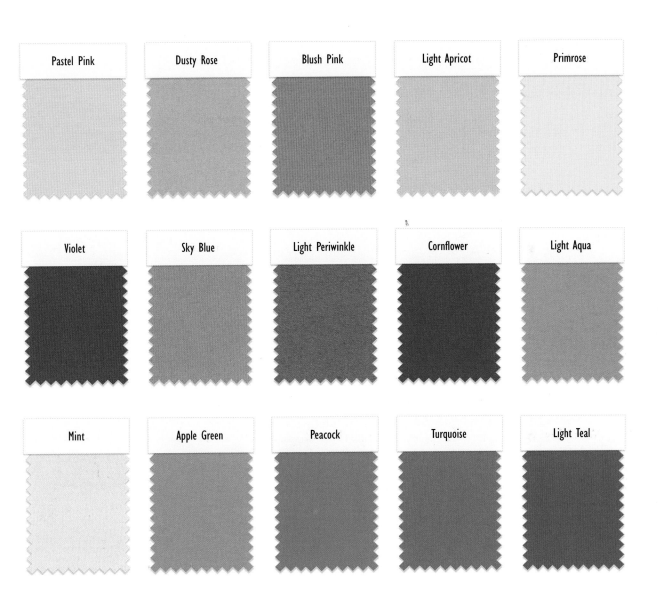

Pastel Pink	Dusty Rose	Blush Pink	Light Apricot	Primrose
Violet	Sky Blue	Light Periwinkle	Cornflower	Light Aqua
Mint	Apple Green	Peacock	Turquoise	Light Teal

LIGHT 1

Women in their twenties with Light coloring have the most delicate look. This youthful, feminine look will often work to your advantage; however, in the work place it may work against you as people may think you are younger than you are. Learning to use the colors in your palette to establish your credibility is the key.

YOUR COLORS

As a youthful Light you will be able to wear the stronger colors from your palette together or in contrast with paler or more muted shades. The wide choice of aquas and greens will give you some great alternatives to the blues, which no doubt you already enjoy wearing. Wear reds and corals with confidence but avoid dark burgundies as these are too overpowering for your coloring. The light shades of grays and navies are ideal for your formal workwear whereas rose brown, taupe, and cocoa are great investment buys.

YOUR HAIR

As a natural blonde your hair will fade or darken in the winter; a dose of sunshine or some blonde highlights will restore your natural blondness.

ACCESSORIZING YOUR LOOK

Try and avoid the black handbag–shoe combination as these will stand out against the lighter shades in your wardrobe. Tan, gray, navies are good basic shades, however do not forget that a colorful handbag will often liven up an outfit as will shoes and scarves.

YOUR MAKEUP

Wherever you are or whatever the weather is, you must always wear a sunscreen to protect your delicate skin against light and sun damage. Although fashion may dictate strong deep colors, these shades will make you look tired and over made-up. Your makeup colors reflect the colors of your palette; as a youthful Light the granite pencil will give you the eye definition that you require.

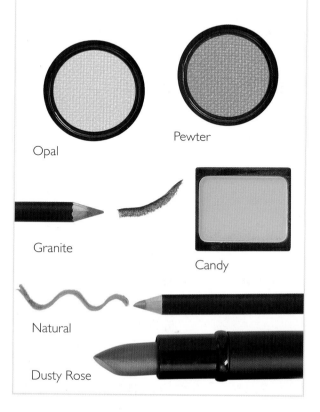

Opal

Pewter

Granite

Candy

Natural

Dusty Rose

YOUR COLOR COMBINATIONS

These color combinations can be used as block colors or in a print.

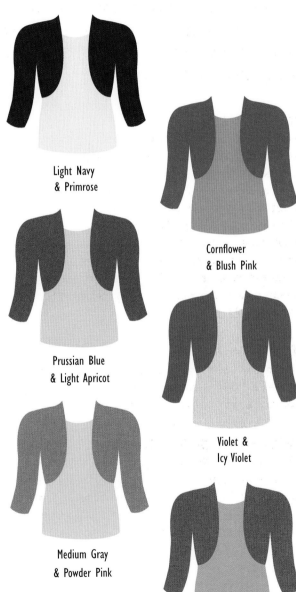

Light Navy
& Primrose

Cornflower
& Blush Pink

Prussian Blue
& Light Apricot

Violet &
Icy Violet

Medium Gray
& Powder Pink

Rose Brown
& Light Aqua

YOUR ADDITIONAL COLORS

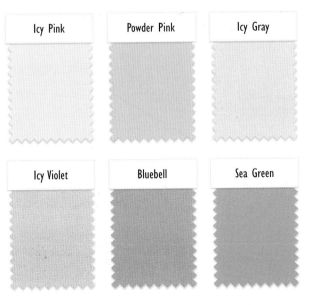

Icy Pink	Powder Pink	Icy Gray

Icy Violet	Bluebell	Sea Green

LIGHT 2

As you mature, you may find that your coloring starts to fade a little and you will fit into our second category of Light. Your coloring will really work to your advantage, particularly if you have looked after your skin, and have kept your youthful appearance. You should now have the confidence to wear the colors that work best for you.

YOUR COLORS

As your natural coloring fades a little you might find it more flattering to wear color combinations that are slightly more muted or you can use colors in a monochromatic way, such as different shades of blues. The fresh tones of apple and yellow-green perfectly complement the softer shades of pewter, cocoa, and taupe. Black is a staple in many women's wardrobes, but you really have to wear it sparingly: below the waist is fine. Your alternative to the LBD (little black dress) is perhaps purple, teal, or even red. If no alternative to black can be found, the fabric should be light and sheer—think chiffon or lace.

YOUR HAIR

Your hair may have noticeably started to fade and it would certainly be a great idea to keep the lightness in your hair by highlighting it. Do avoid ash tones, however, as these will not be flattering with the colors of your color palette.

ACCESSORIZING YOUR LOOK

If the time has come that you need to wear glasses on a more regular basis, you need to choose frames that are either light in color or in construction. Make sure that your earrings do not conflict with your glasses.

YOUR MAKEUP

Now may be the time to consider such beauty treatments as tinting your eyelashes and eyebrows to keep some definition, as the use of cosmetics to achieve this can become heavy and overpowering. Use a warm brown mascara, which will be more flattering than a black one.

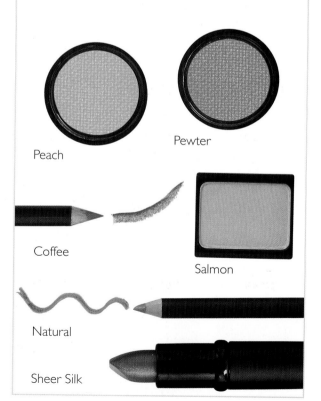

Peach

Pewter

Coffee

Salmon

Natural

Sheer Silk

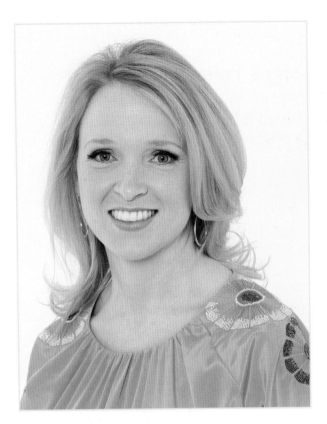

YOUR ADDITIONAL COLORS

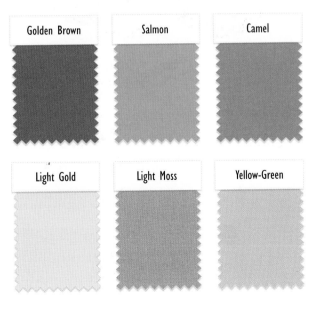

| Golden Brown | Salmon | Camel |
| Light Gold | Light Moss | Yellow-Green |

YOUR COLOR COMBINATIONS

These color combinations can be used as block colors or in a print.

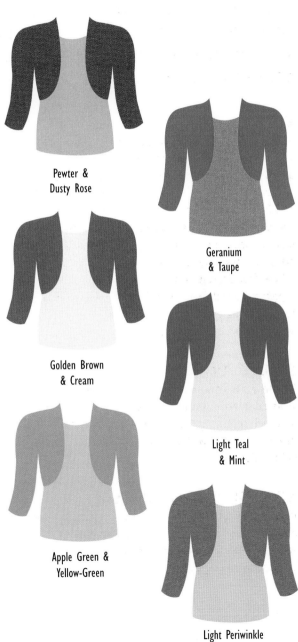

Pewter &
Dusty Rose

Geranium
& Taupe

Golden Brown
& Cream

Light Teal
& Mint

Apple Green &
Yellow-Green

Light Periwinkle
& Light Apricot

LIGHT 3

As this third type of Light, you may have been a Light all your life but as you have matured your hair color has lightened, your eye color has paled, and your skin tone has become more delicate. Now is the right time to re-evaluate your look and the colors that you wear to ensure you keep that spring in your step.

YOUR COLORS

As a maturing Light you need to wear colors that are slightly stronger than those you may have worn in the past, since you may have lost some of your clarity. Your neutral shades can be worn on their own or mixed with other shades in a print or a weave. Add a pop of color (vest, scarf, or top) if you choose to wear a more tonal look. If you choose to wear the darker shades of your palette (say, light navy or Prussian blue) be sure to wear a pale color under the chin (no one wants dark shadows reflecting on the face).

YOUR HAIR

Continue to tint or highlight your hair; however, you have the option to stay with nature and go white within the spectrum of the Light coloring. Often people with your coloring have fine hair, so use products to add volume.

ACCESSORIZING YOUR LOOK

Adding jewelry will enhance your look. Make sure that the colors are within the framework of your color palette and do not overpower you. A stunning brooch, or pair of earrings, will draw attention away from a not-so-perfect neck, while a long necklace is a great alternative to one that is choker style.

YOUR MAKEUP

You will benefit from wearing a foundation rather than a tinted moisturizer. Keep powdering but only on the bony parts of the face (forehead, nose, cheeks, and chin). Matte eye shadows and lipsticks are more flattering than anything with frost and glitter. Tinting your eyebrows and eyelashes is now a must in order to flatter your eyes.

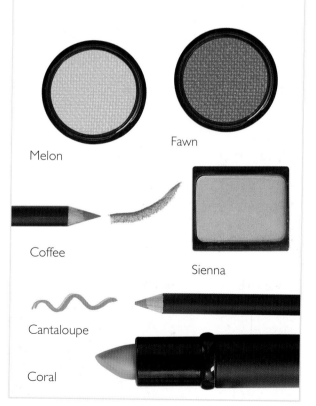

Melon

Fawn

Coffee

Sienna

Cantaloupe

Coral

YOUR COLOR COMBINATIONS

These color combinations can be used as block colors or in a print.

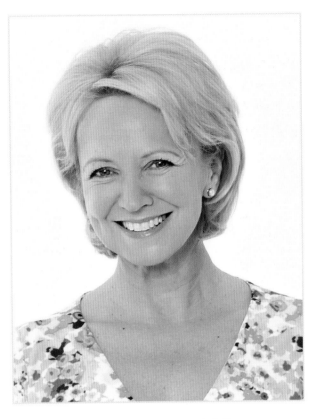

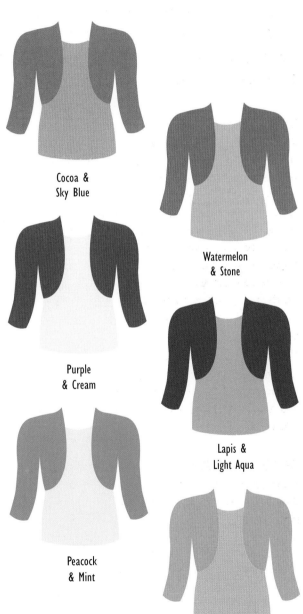

Cocoa &
Sky Blue

Watermelon
& Stone

Purple
& Cream

Lapis &
Light Aqua

Peacock
& Mint

Coral Pink
& Light Gray

YOUR ADDITIONAL COLORS

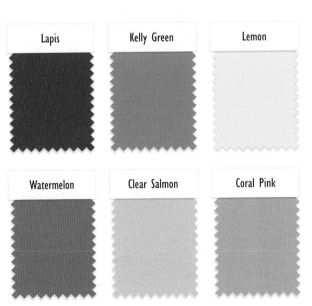

Lapis	Kelly Green	Lemon

Watermelon	Clear Salmon	Coral Pink

ARE YOU A DEEP ?

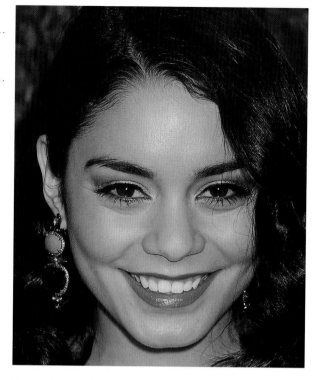

Vanessa Hudgens has a strong look with brown eyes and dark brown hair color, which is enhanced with a bright red lipstick.

DO YOU HAVE ...

- Dark brown to black hair?
- Dark eyes?
- Dark eyebrows and lashes?
- Skin tone from porcelain to dark brown or black, including all the shades in between?

YOUR LOOK IS

- Dark and strong.
- The undertone of your skin may be either warm or cool.
- Your overall look is deep.
- You may be clear or soft.

YOUR IDEAL COLORS

For a master color palette: go to pages 64–65.

HOW TO WEAR YOUR COLORS

You can wear black on its own, or team it with dark shades such as black-brown and eggplant for day or royal purple for a sophisticated look. If you are a Dramatic type (see pages 28–29), try black with a single bold color such as scarlet.

To balance your look, wear strong, dark colors near your face. Contrast these with lighter or brighter shades from your palette. Wear two dark colors, or light and dark, but never wear two light colors together.

BE AWARE

In a warmer climate you may be tempted to go for lighter shades, but be careful when wearing pale or pastel shades on their own. These will always look better on you when worn with dark or bright colors for contrast. Be bold and choose brighter colors from your palette such as lime, emerald green, turquoise, or blush pink, and combine them with stone or taupe. Remember to wear the stronger colors near your face. If you decide to wear light shades near your face, balance your look with deeper-colored makeup so that you don't look pale and washed out.

BEING A DEEP

There are many differing types of Deeps as shown with our celebrities. All have the same strong look of dark hair and deep strong eyes with skin tones ranging from porcelain to dark brown. Differences in skin tone and eye color will give some variation in the additional colors

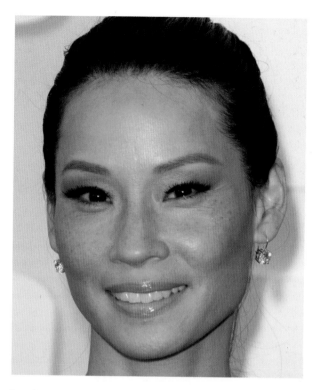

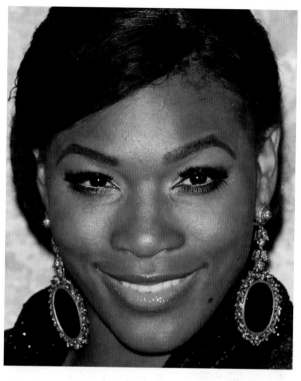

Lucy Liu has black hair with an olive skin tone and brown eyes, giving her a striking Deep appearance.

Serena Williams has a dark brown skin tone, dark brown eyes and dark brown hair, which completes the picture of a stunning Deep.

shown on the following pages. If a few gray hairs appear, consider tinting your hair to keep your deep appearance.

TIPS FOR WEARING YOUR COLORS

The key to being Deep and wearing your colors successfully is that you can wear two dark colors together, light and dark or just a dark color on its own. If this does not work for you, then you are not a Deep; refer to the Clear or Soft colorings to see if you fit there. As the colors in your palette are rather strong it is important that you balance your look with the appropriate makeup for your color type. Look through the following pages and see the recommended colors for your particular type; pale lipsticks might be fashionable but they will not be your best look.

COLORING YOUR HAIR

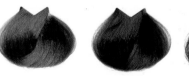

| Brown | Dark brown | Deep dark brown |

To qualify as any of our Deep types you must have dark brown or black hair, which may have either warm or cool tones to it.

DEEP COLOR PALETTE

INVESTMENT COLORS

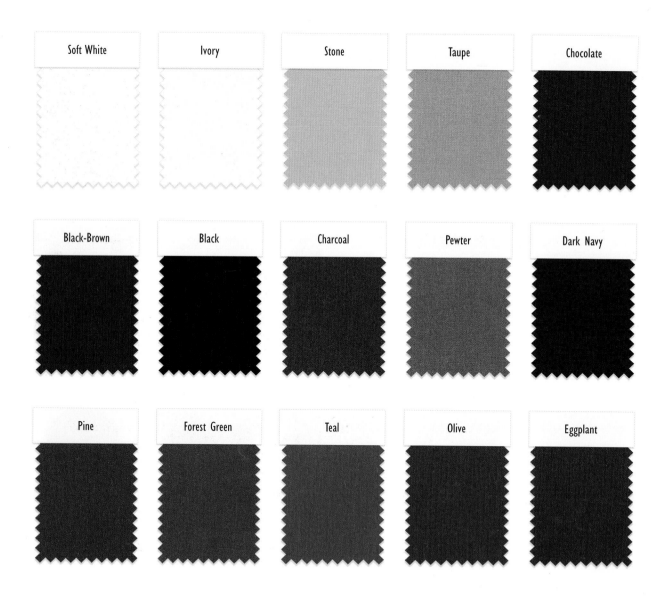

| Soft White | Ivory | Stone | Taupe | Chocolate |

| Black-Brown | Black | Charcoal | Pewter | Dark Navy |

| Pine | Forest Green | Teal | Olive | Eggplant |

FASHION COLORS

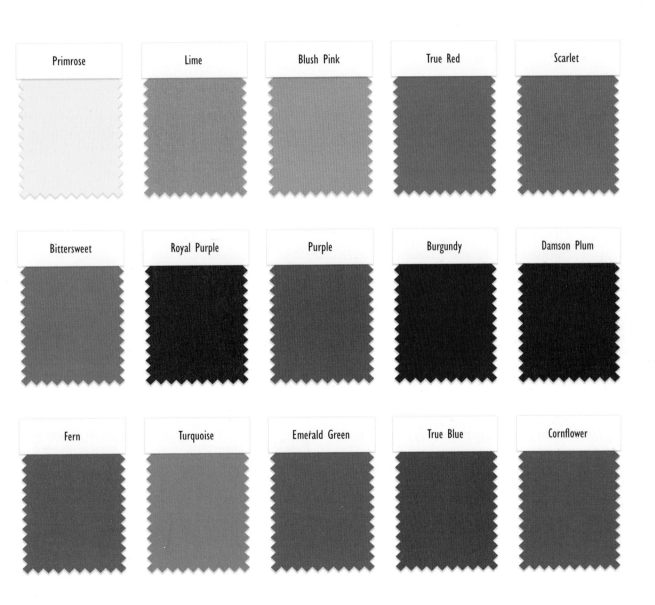

Primrose	Lime	Blush Pink	True Red	Scarlet
Bittersweet	Royal Purple	Purple	Burgundy	Damson Plum
Fern	Turquoise	Emerald Green	True Blue	Cornflower

DEEP 1

This look is dominated by dark hair and deep eyes, and you fit into this first category of Deep if you have a pale to olive skin tone. Depending on your lifestyle and style personality, you may need to tweak how you put your wardrobe together so as not to create an overpowering appearance. Use your light shades with dark contrast.

YOUR COLORS

Black is a color that you may wear head to toe. Do not forget, however, that on occasion you can soften the look by adding a lighter shade; think ivory, primrose, lime, or salmon. Olive is another versatile color that can be worn for your casual and workwear. Browns will always be stunning on you, and when you want to add a brighter look to your wardrobe true blue, cornflower, and purple are just wonderful. In the summer, if you are wearing taupe or stone, add a contrasting shade such as true red, turquoise, or blush pink.

YOUR HAIR

Deeps have a tendency to gray prematurely. If you want to stay Deep you will need to tint your hair or add lowlights. If you embrace your gray hair coming through, there will be a time when you will have to consider being a Cool or Soft.

ACCESSORIZING YOUR LOOK

Against the deep colors of your wardrobe, you can use contrasting colors for your accessories. Darker and heavier frames for your glasses will be best.

YOUR MAKEUP

The strength of your palette requires you to take particular care with your makeup. You need bold makeup to balance your strong and rich look with the deep colors of your palette. A red lipstick will be stunning on you: try tomato or ruby which will be more flattering than a bright crimson.

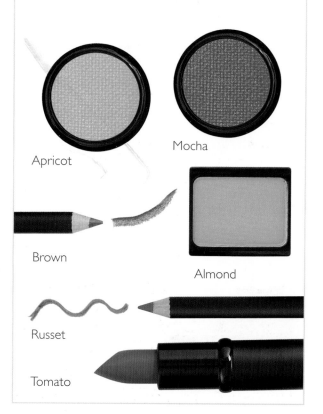

Apricot

Mocha

Brown

Almond

Russet

Tomato

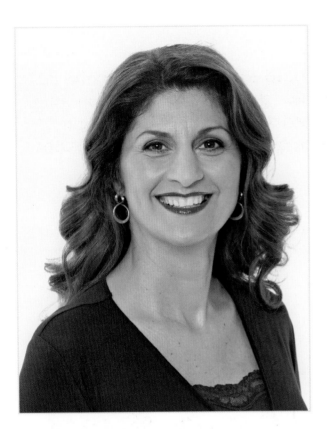

YOUR COLOR COMBINATIONS

These color combinations can be used as block colors or in a print.

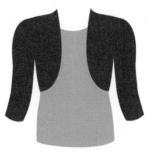

Forest Green
& Salmon

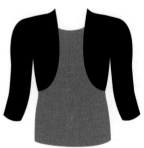

Black
& Moss

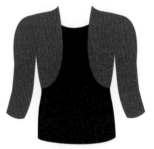

Rust &
Chocolate

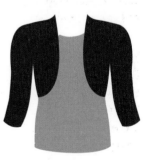

Damson Plum
& Camel

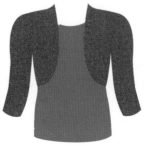

Pewter &
Bittersweet

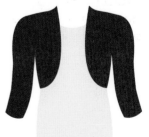

Olive &
Primrose

YOUR ADDITIONAL COLORS

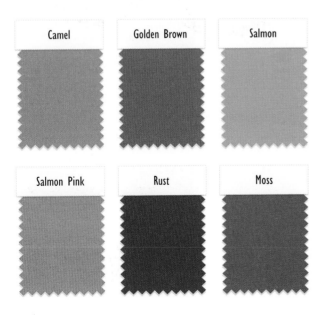

Camel	Golden Brown	Salmon
Salmon Pink	Rust	Moss

DEEP 2

As this second type of Deep you have golden tones to your skin, rather than olive; your dark eyes have a slight clarity to them as the whites of your eyes are more defined; and your hair is dark. You will wear your colors in a bolder fashion and focus your colors on those rich, warm, and deep shades such as pumpkin and tomato red.

YOUR COLORS

Vibrant, rich colors will be the mainstay of your wardrobe. When using your neutrals, add a contrasting color or a light shade. Black and soft white is a great combination and never goes out of fashion. Chocolate and ivory is an interesting alternative. All the shades of red in your palette will be great energizing colors. In warmer climates use turquoise, lime, true blue, and cornflower to create a stunning look.

YOUR HAIR

As with all types of Deep, it is essential to keep your hair dark. If you opt to color your hair, use dark brown or dark golden brown. Lowlights will also work for you, but do not go more than one shade lighter than your natural hair color.

ACCESSORIZING YOUR LOOK

Statement earrings are a great way of drawing attention to your face; make sure that any stones and metals reflect the colors of your palette. Your shoe color should be at least as dark or darker than your hemline—a light-colored pair of shoes with dark pants or skirts never looks good.

YOUR MAKEUP

With this particular coloring you need to avoid pinky shades of foundations, which will not sit well with your natural skin tone. Your eyes will look incredible with rich colored tones of peppermint and a teal pencil. Your deep colored eyes will always benefit from lashings of mascara—you may also want to use an eyelash curler. Don't forget to enhance the color of your eyebrows, if these are starting to fade.

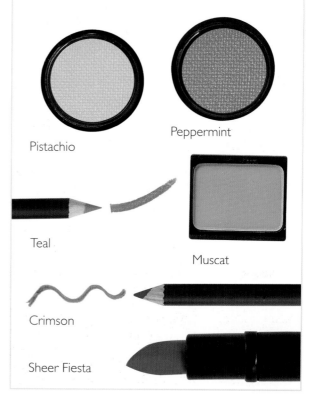

Pistachio

Peppermint

Teal

Muscat

Crimson

Sheer Fiesta

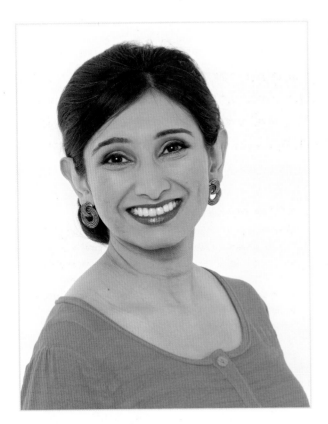

YOUR COLOR COMBINATIONS

These color combinations can be used as block colors or in a print.

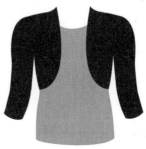

Charcoal
& Mustard

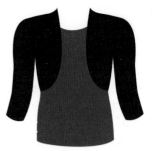

Black-Brown
& Evergreen

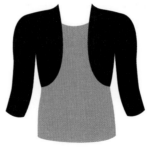

Dark Navy
& Lime

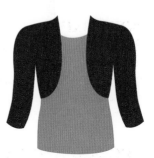

Pine
& Pumpkin

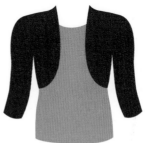

Royal Purple
& Blush Pink

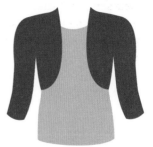

True Blue
& Stone

YOUR ADDITIONAL COLORS

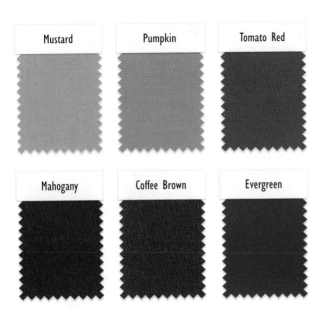

Mustard	Pumpkin	Tomato Red
Mahogany	Coffee Brown	Evergreen

DEEP 3

Our third type of Deep's look is stunning. There is a wonderful balance between the depth of your hair color, your dark brown skin tone, and your deep eye color. Your one challenge is that you do not look good in pale shades, ever, and consequently you really need to focus on the darker colors to be found in your palette.

YOUR COLORS

Wearing two dark colors from your palette is probably the easiest and most successful way to combine colors for this coloring type. To achieve a more interesting look, and break away from wearing the traditional black, think about chocolate brown, pine, or even eggplant or burgundy. To lighten the look, you may add a lighter shade from your palette by adding a T-shirt/tank in an ivory, soft white, primrose, or lime. Always make sure you have one of your darker shades near the face (think jacket, sweater, shirt).

YOUR HAIR

Depending on your hair type you may wish to keep it natural looking, consider wearing one of the many wonderful wigs available, or have hair extensions put in. Beware that if you drastically change your hair color, you may no longer be Deep and could become a Soft 3 (see pages 110–111).

ACCESSORIZING YOUR LOOK

Against your dark skin nothing looks more stunning than a deep bright shade of nail color (don't forget your toes). Use your fashion colors (see page 65) in scarves, shawls, and pashminas to bring some excitement to your wardrobe.

YOUR MAKEUP

Matching your foundation to your skin tone might be a challenge for someone with dark skin as you may have slight color variation in your skin. Consider using two different shades of foundation in the appropriate areas to give an overall even appearance. Use a bronzer for shading rather than a blush. Fuller lips always look better with deeper nonfrosted shades of lipstick.

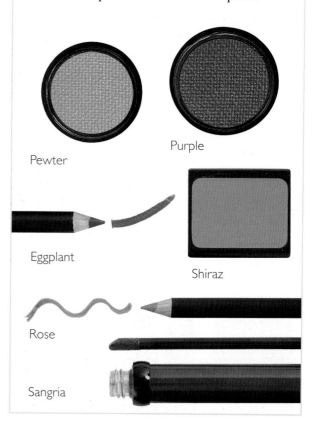

Pewter

Purple

Eggplant

Shiraz

Rose

Sangria

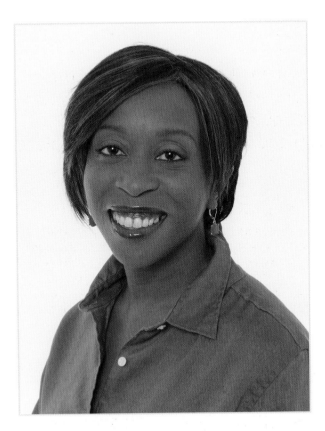

YOUR ADDITIONAL COLORS

Dark Teal	Lavender	Violet

Plum	Fuchsia	Raspberry

YOUR COLOR COMBINATIONS

These color combinations can be used as block colors or in a print.

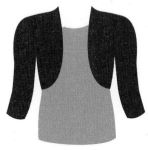

Eggplant & Lavender

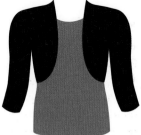

Black & Raspberry

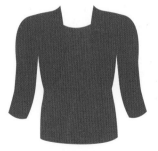

Plum & Purple

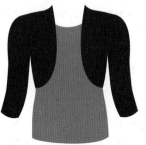

Black-Brown & Scarlet

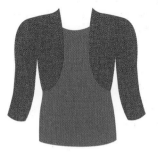

Pewter & Fern

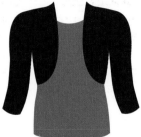

Dark Navy & Cornflower

ARE YOU A WARM ?

DO YOU HAVE ...

- Red-toned hair in any shade from strawberry blonde to auburn?
- Green, brown, or blue eyes?
- Eyebrows in a warm tone, from reddish to brown?
- Blonde to dark eyelashes?
- Porcelain skin, possibly with an abundance of freckles, or darker-toned skin with a golden glow to it?

YOUR LOOK IS

- Warm and golden.
- The undertone of your skin is warm.
- Your overall look is medium in depth.
- You may be either clear or soft.

YOUR IDEAL COLORS

For a master color palette: go to pages 74–75.

HOW TO WEAR YOUR COLORS

Because your overall look is warm, the golden rule is to balance it by choosing colors that have a warm (yellow) undertone. You will always look best in colors that are medium in depth, rather than light or deep. When wearing navy or gray, warm them up with tones of yellow, salmon, or peach.

BE AWARE

As your look is warm and golden, don't be tempted to buy items in baby pink or icy violet, as these colors will make you look gray. When wearing the darker neutrals in your palette, try to balance them with the lighter or paler shades, as your overall look should

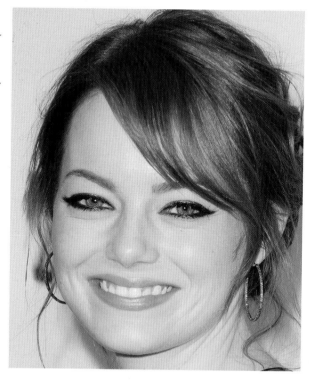

Emma Stone has a pale porcelain skin tone, complementary blue eyes, and auburn hair that make her a wonderful Warm type.

be medium in depth. Keep makeup colors warm, especially blusher and lipstick. Salmon and peachy shades will make you come alive. Avoid using black mascara and eyeliner.

BEING A WARM

The main attribute to being a Warm, as you can see from the celebrity pictures here, is that the key features have a warm undertone to them. Your hair must have red tones to it, be it a strawberry blonde or deep rich auburn. Skin tones, whether pale porcelain or golden brown, will often feature freckles and will look golden. The eyes will be green, brown, or even blue, but blue eyes will often have yellow or green flecks in them. When any gray or white hairs start to appear consider

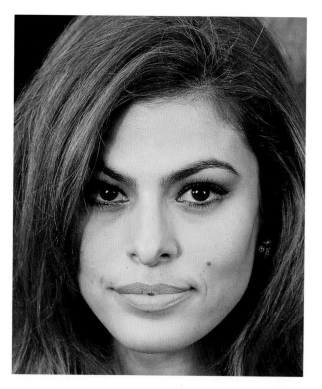

Eva Mendes has a warm skin tone, stunning brown eyes, and ivory skin, giving her an overall golden glow.

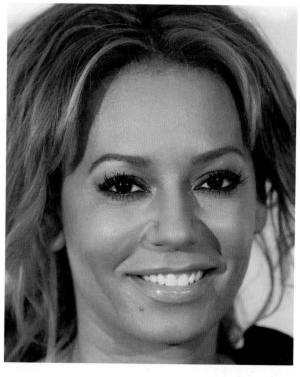

Mel B has the deepest look of our celebrities, with a darker skin tone, auburn hair, and dark brown eyes.

tinting your hair with warm tones or lowlights to keep the basic tones warm; if you start to have more than 50 percent gray you may need to change your palette.

TIPS FOR WEARING YOUR COLORS

All your colors need to have a yellow or warm tone to them. The deeper your hair color the stronger you can go with your colors. Those of you with porcelain skin tone and strawberry blonde hair need to ensure you put lighter shades with your gray and navy. It is hard for many women to give up wearing black but if you have it in your wardrobe, use accessories and makeup to warm the look up. Any gold or copper metals will be great, or choose warm colors from your palette as colors for necklaces or scarves.

COLORING YOUR HAIR

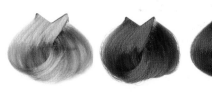

Strawberry blonde   Auburn   Deep copper

Always keep your warm tones, whether you decide to go lighter or darker. If you start to gray prematurely, use an overall warm tint, otherwise you will change your dominant color type.

WARM COLOR PALETTE

INVESTMENT COLORS

Soft White	Cream	Stone	Taupe	Oatmeal

Bronze	Pewter	Charcoal	Chocolate	Light Navy

Teal	Olive	Gray-Green	Sage	Purple

FASHION COLORS

Mint	Primrose	Daffodil	Tangerine	Amber
Lime	Apricot	Terracotta	Orange-Red	Bittersweet
Coral	True Red	Light Periwinkle	Aqua	Turquoise

WARM 1

If you have porcelain skin with strawberry blonde hair you have a typical Warm coloring. Your green eyes will be complemented by the warm tones of your color palette. This first type of Warm will often be covered in freckles and have a sensitive skin that burns easily in the sun. Make sure your foundation has a sunscreen or wear one underneath.

YOUR COLORS

As with all Warms, you need to ensure that all your colors have a yellow undertone. When wearing light navy or charcoal gray, make sure you add a warm-toned top near your face such as peach, primrose, or coral. Beware when choosing your pinks that you are not tempted by pretty baby pinks and fuchsias. Blues are not a big feature in your wardrobe; concentrate instead on your aquas and periwinkles. With your pale, translucent skin, avoid wearing two dark colors together because this combination will overpower your delicate look.

YOUR HAIR

Use a golden tint when the natural gray highlights start to appear. Don't be tempted to go darker as darker hair will look harsh against your porcelain skin. If you want to add color, copper or strawberry highlights will work best for you.

ACCESSORIZING YOUR LOOK

Your choice of jewelry is determined by your warm tones. Try creamy or apricot-toned pearls, especially when worn with your neutrals. If you wear glasses—and sunglasses—consider the color of your frames as you want these to blend with your warm look.

YOUR MAKEUP

Make sure your foundation really blends with your skin color and don't attempt to hide those freckles (also known as angels' kisses), they are part of your look. Before settling on eye shadow shades, check your palette to make sure that they are of a similar tone, and at all costs avoid blue-based lipstick or blusher because these will look harsh and unnatural on you.

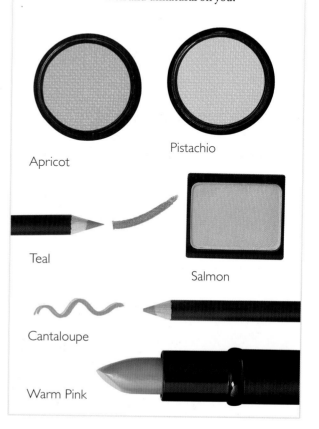

Apricot

Pistachio

Teal

Salmon

Cantaloupe

Warm Pink

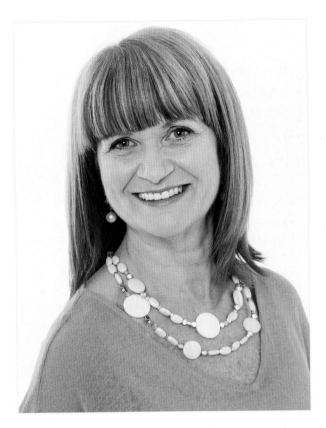

YOUR COLOR COMBINATIONS

These color combinations can be used as block colors or in a print.

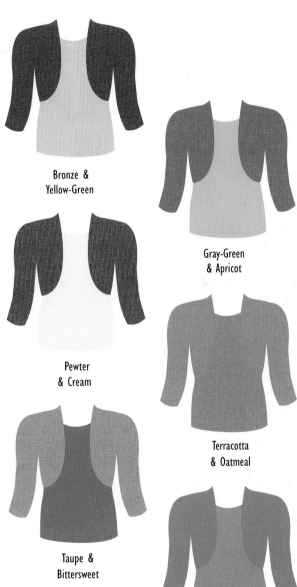

Bronze & Yellow-Green

Gray-Green & Apricot

Pewter & Cream

Terracotta & Oatmeal

Taupe & Bittersweet

Turquoise & Aqua

YOUR ADDITIONAL COLORS

Buttermilk	Light Peach	Peach

Light Gold	Yellow-Green	Light Moss

WARM 2

If you choose to add warm and vibrant tones to your hair to give yourself a dramatic fashion appearance, your skin tone is light to medium in depth, and you have green or light brown eyes, you fit into our second category of Warm. You will look fantastic in rich and warm colors. And don't forget to balance your look with some vibrant makeup colors.

YOUR COLORS

Your look is rather exotic and with your strength of coloring you can wear a wonderful array of color combinations and take your inspiration from baroque and Moroccan hues. Do not shy away from wearing your darker colors together: try bittersweet, lime, or terracotta with chocolate or purple. For more formal wear, try charcoal with apricot or coral. In warmer climates, rather than wearing pale shades, try the hot vibrant colors from your palette like amber, daffodil, or aqua. When wearing the lighter shades such as mint, primrose, and cream, complement them with light navy, teal, or bronze in a print, or an interesting textured fabric.

YOUR HAIR

Add rich, warm gold or copper tones to enhance the richness of the color of your hair. When natural gray highlights appear, cover them with a copper or red tint or a henna treatment.

ACCESSORIZING YOUR LOOK

When building your neutral wardrobe try bronze, tan, and brown shoes and handbags to complement your warm tones. For something a little more colorful think tangerine, amber, or lime accessories. Gold and warm-colored beads either in jewelry or as embellishment will complete your look.

YOUR MAKEUP

When applying your eye makeup, warm smoky eyes will be a great glamour look; for everyday don't forget to use your eyeliner to give definition to your beautiful eyes, even if this is all you do on a daily basis. If you are not elaborating on the eye makeup, you will need a stronger warm-toned lipstick to balance your look.

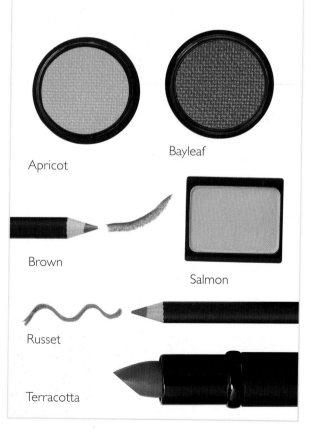

Apricot

Bayleaf

Brown

Salmon

Russet

Terracotta

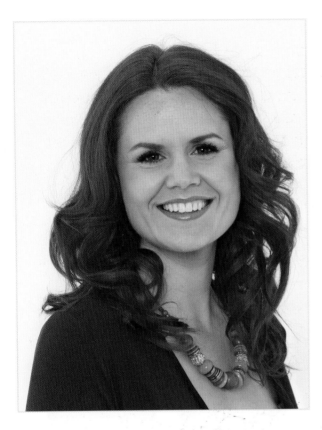

YOUR COLOR COMBINATIONS

These color combinations can be used as block colors or in a print.

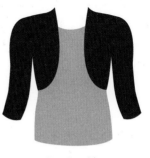

Chocolate &
Coral Pink

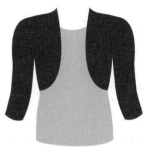

Olive &
Apricot

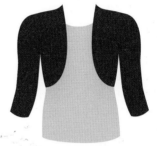

Charcoal
& Daffodil

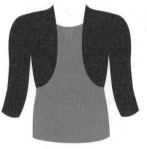

Teal &
Turquoise

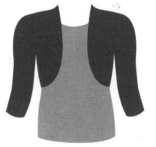

Bittersweet
& Sage

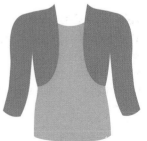

Kelly Green
& Amber

YOUR ADDITIONAL COLORS

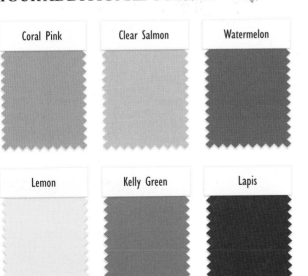

Coral Pink	Clear Salmon	Watermelon
Lemon	Kelly Green	Lapis

WARM 3

As this third type of Warm you have naturally auburn or reddish hair, your skin tone is of medium depth, and you have an abundance of freckles. Anyone who has dark or golden skin and freckles should consider themselves part of this category. This look can be created by tinting your hair if it was dark and is now lighter.

YOUR COLORS

The medium tones in your wardrobe will perfectly balance with your look. You have the choice, depending on your lifestyle and your personality, to either make it a tone-on-tone look or use colors in a more dramatic way. For a tone-on-tone look use colors such as olive and moss, golden brown and chocolate, or rust with salmon pink. For a more dramatic look why not try aqua with lime, or daffodil and purple. Your warm reds will go brilliantly when you combine them with oatmeal, sage, and even terracotta.

YOUR HAIR

The warm golden tones of your hair will naturally complement your warm skin tone, so make sure you keep your hair in peak condition to enhance its natural shine and color.

ACCESSORIZING YOUR LOOK

When it comes to jewelry, natural materials are great for you as well as metals like copper, bronze, and of course gold. Great colors for semiprecious stones are jade, topaz, amber, peridot, coral, and aquamarine. Think about bringing colors and textures to your outfits in the form of scarves, hats, and gloves.

YOUR MAKEUP

If you find it difficult to match a foundation to your skin tone consider using a tinted moisturizer, which will allow your gorgeous freckles to shine through. If you are on the mature side, you will need to use a foundation to give you a more even complexion. Shades of copper and coral lipstick will enhance your natural coloring and a brown mascara is more flattering than a black one.

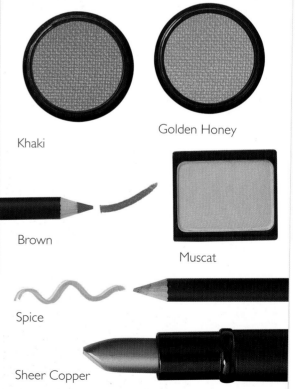

Khaki

Golden Honey

Brown

Muscat

Spice

Sheer Copper

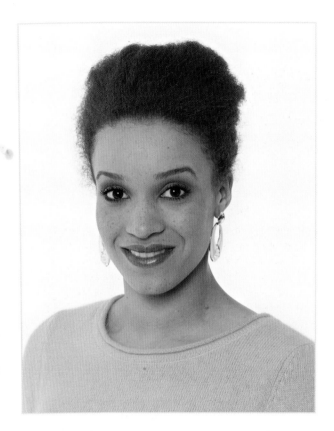

YOUR COLOR COMBINATIONS

These color combinations can be used as block colors or in a print.

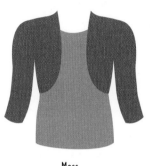

Moss
& Lime

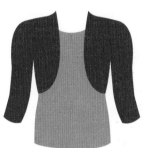

Rust &
Tangerine

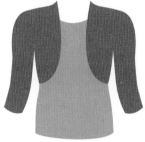

Golden Brown
& Salmon

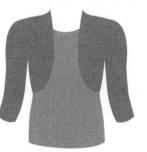

Light Periwinkle
& Camel

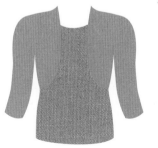

Coral &
Taupe

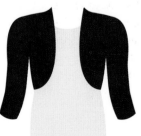

Light Navy
& Primrose

YOUR ADDITIONAL COLORS

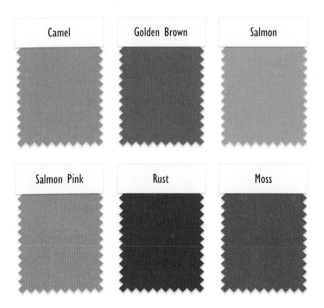

Camel	Golden Brown	Salmon

Salmon Pink	Rust	Moss

ARE YOU A COOL ?

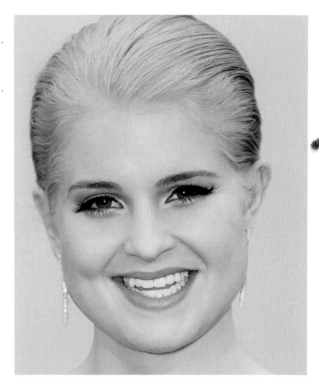

Kelly Osbourne is one of many young woman who tint their hair ash or gray tones and it works with pink-toned skin coloring.

DO YOU HAVE ...
- Ash tones to your hair, be it dark brown, blonde, white, or gray?
- Gray, blue, green, or clear brown eyes?
- Eyebrows and eyelashes that range in color from the lighter shade of blonde to dark brown?
- Pink undertones to your skin or porcelain skin that appears transluscent? A dark brown or black skin may have a slight blue tinge.

YOUR LOOK IS
- Cool and pinkish.
- The undertone of your skin is cool.
- The overall depth of your coloring is medium to deep.
- The clarity of your look may be either clear or soft.

YOUR IDEAL COLORS
For a master color palette: go to pages 84–85.

HOW TO WEAR YOUR COLORS
Because your look is cool and pinkish, all your colors need to have a cool (blue) undertone, preferably with some contrast. You will always look best in medium to deep colors. If you wear brown, balance it with cool shades from your palette, such as teal or rose pink.

BE AWARE
Avoid colors that have a warm, yellow tone, as these will make your skin appear sallow. If you do wear yellow, make it as a print. Browns need to have a pinky, rather than yellow, tone. When wearing your darker neutrals, balance them with the lighter and brighter shades from your color chart and avoid wearing two dark neutrals together. Keep all your makeup colors cool and beware of brown-based lipsticks, especially pale, natural-looking shades.

BEING COOL
Some women are born with cool coloring, others become cool as they mature. To be Cool there has to be a complete lack of any warm tones in the hair and eye color. Cool skin tones can be rosy pink or absolute porcelain skin that looks translucent, while anyone with dark brown or black skin will appear to have a blue or even gray tinge to it. Cools with pink or rosy skin tones will often need to use brighter shades, as they have lost

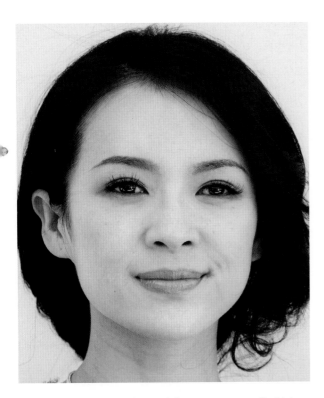

Zhang Ziyi's striking porcelain cool skin contrasts so well with her blue-black hair and stunning, deep brown eyes.

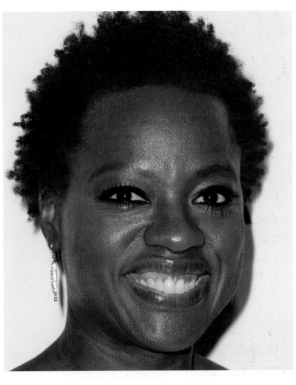

Viola Davis has a wonderful blue-black skin tone, very dark brown eyes and dark brown hair ensuring her cool coloring.

some definition, whereas those with porcelain skin and black hair already have a lot of contrast in their look. If your hair is salt and pepper you may not be Cool, it will depend on the percentage of white you have. If it is more than 60 percent white, you may still be Cool, but if not, refer to the Soft palette.

TIPS FOR WEARING YOUR COLORS

All the colors you wear should have a cool or blue base to them. Black is in your palette, but is best worn with some contrast or in a sheer fabric, especially near the face. As gray or silver hair is becoming more fashionable, pink and purple tones are being added. These are fun, but make sure the rest of your look goes with this fashion statement.

COLORING YOUR HAIR

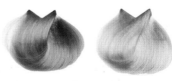

Ash   Silver   Black

Cool hair tones vary from pure white to most shades of gray, cool dark brown, and all the way to an ebony type of black, as well as salt and pepper.

COOL COLOR PALETTE

INVESTMENT COLORS

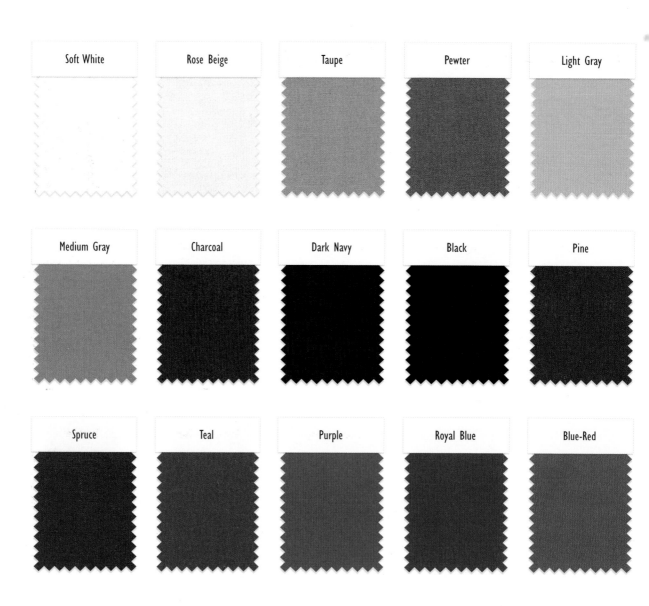

Soft White	Rose Beige	Taupe	Pewter	Light Gray

Medium Gray	Charcoal	Dark Navy	Black	Pine

Spruce	Teal	Purple	Royal Blue	Blue-Red

FASHION COLORS

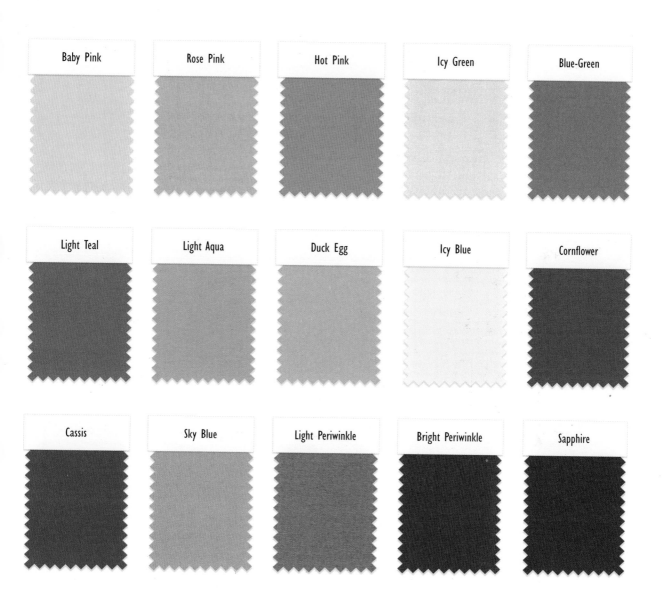

| Baby Pink | Rose Pink | Hot Pink | Icy Green | Blue-Green |

| Light Teal | Light Aqua | Duck Egg | Icy Blue | Cornflower |

| Cassis | Sky Blue | Light Periwinkle | Bright Periwinkle | Sapphire |

COOL 1

More and more women are embracing going "gray" prematurely. Often having a silver mane will be a fashion statement—as demonstrated by the likes of Helen Mirren and Kelly Osbourne. You are our first type of Cool if you have blue eyes and rosy pink tones to your skin. If you decide to go gray this will mean revamping your wardrobe and makeup shades.

YOUR COLORS

The cool palette has a wide variation of both light and dark colors, as well as clear and soft colors. The best color combination for this type of Cool is either to use the lighter brighter colors in the palette or, when wearing your darker shades, to do so with a lighter color. Although black is in the palette, soften it with paler shades such as baby pink, icy violet, or sky blue. If you are unsure about wearing red, texture will soften its appearance, but you will still benefit from its energetic and dramatic effect. Be warned that wearing all your "sweet pea" colors (icy violet, bluebell, baby pink) together will have an ageing effect. Those colors are great, but use them in contrast with darker colors or as part of a print.

YOUR HAIR

If you hair is ash blonde you will gray gracefully but make sure that any highlights or color you put into your hair is ash- or platinum-based for a seamless transition. Avoid any red tints.

ACCESSORIZING YOUR LOOK

For shoes and handbags, navy is the safest combination to wear with all your cool colors, but do not forget that a splash of color will update your look. Your watch is also an accessory, so make it work for your palette, and demonstrate how "trendy" you are.

YOUR MAKEUP

The overall look of your makeup should be cool, using blue-based shades to balance your dominant coloring; this includes your lipstick and blush colors. If your eyebrows have lost their color, perhaps consider tinting them or use an eyebrow pencil.

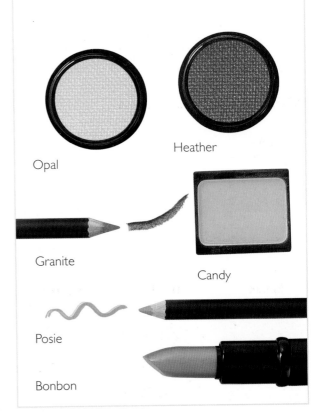

Opal

Heather

Granite

Candy

Posie

Bonbon

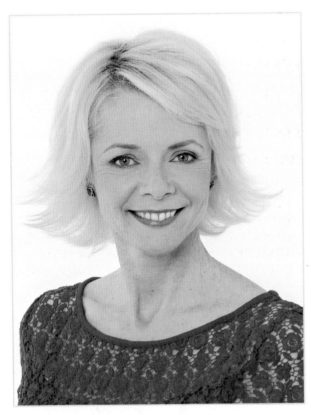

YOUR COLOR COMBINATIONS

These color combinations can be used as block colors or in a print.

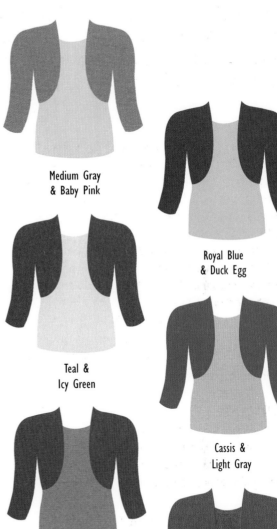

Medium Gray & Baby Pink

Royal Blue & Duck Egg

Teal & Icy Green

Cassis & Light Gray

Bright Periwinkle & Light Periwinkle

Blue-Red & Pewter

YOUR ADDITIONAL COLORS

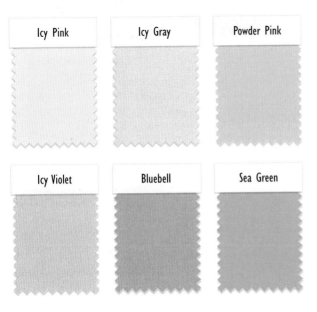

Icy Pink	Icy Gray	Powder Pink

Icy Violet	Bluebell	Sea Green

COOL 2

You fit into our second category of Cool if you have blue-black hair with not a trace of red tone to it; your skin is virtually translucent with an alabaster appearance and a cool tone and your eyes are a striking cool black-brown. Contrast is key to your look whether it is in the color combinations of your clothes or the makeup you choose to wear.

YOUR COLORS

Black and pure white work so well for this type of Cool, which demands a high degree of contrast from light to dark when putting their palette together. When wearing one color, it needs to have depth and contrast, blue, red, bright periwinkle, or royal blue, for example. Pine and spruce are great neutrals but will need to be worn with icy green or icy blue as a contrast. Medium depth neutrals such as pewter and taupe need some vibrancy such as blue-green and cyclamen. In warmer climates, duck egg, light aqua, and hot pink will be striking. When wearing pure white, don't forget a colorful statement accessory.

YOUR HAIR

Cut, color, and condition are the best rules to keep your wonderful head of hair shiny and in control. Avoid the temptation to add any red tones to your hair. As an alternative, try plum, burgundy, or purple lowlights for a bit of fun if you wish.

ACCESSORIZING YOUR LOOK

Depending on your scale, choose your accessories with care (see Scale, pages 138–139). One statement piece will be stunning; think silver, pewter, and platinum for metals, or any color from your palette for stones.

YOUR MAKEUP

Your foundation needs to be the palest of them all, geisha-like. If your skin is free of blemishes, a porcelain powder over your moisturizer may suffice. Depending on your personality you may opt for a bright dramatic red, or for a more subtle look you could choose a deep rose pink or soft mauve.

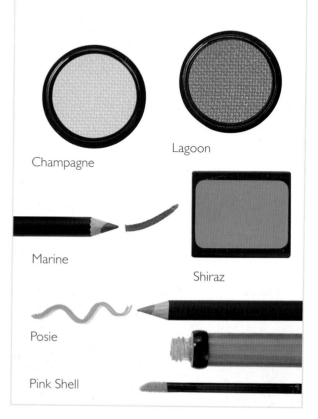

Champagne

Lagoon

Marine

Shiraz

Posie

Pink Shell

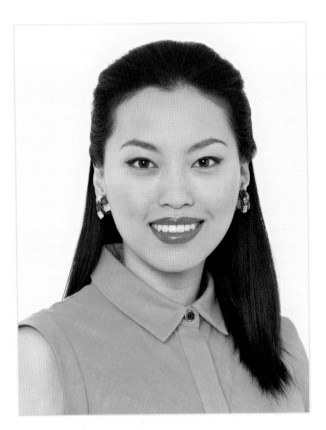

YOUR COLOR COMBINATIONS

These color combinations can be used as block colors or in a print.

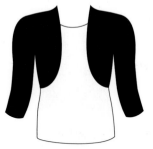

Black &
Pure White

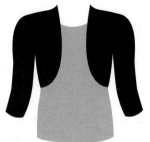

Dark Navy &
Light Aqua

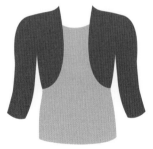

Purple &
Light Gray

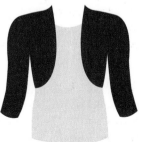

Pine &
Icy Green

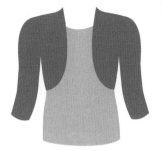

Light Teal
& Rose Pink

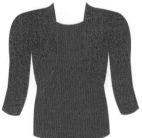

Pewter &
Blue-Red

YOUR ADDITIONAL COLORS

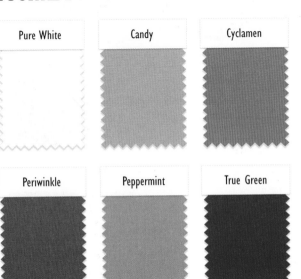

| Pure White | Candy | Cyclamen |
| Periwinkle | Peppermint | True Green |

COOL 3

As this third type of Cool, you may have a darker skin tone with a hint of a blue to it, perhaps best described as rose brown. You also fit into this category if you have very dark brown skin without any warm undertones. Lucky you, though: with your coloring if you start to gray early your color palette will nevertheless remain constant both for your clothes and makeup.

YOUR COLORS

Dark and strong color combinations from within your palette will always be your most striking look. Think black and royal blue, pine and purple, or blue-red and cassis. The light and icy tones in your palette need to be worn with some of the darker shades in your palette. Think icy green with pine, icy blue with cornflower or powder blue with dark navy. The best way for you to wear pewter and taupe is away from the face, or keep these shades as part of a strong print.

YOUR HAIR

As you age, your hair may become a beautiful silver gray or even pure white, which will allow you to then keep the same colored wardrobe. For a fun look, try purple or burgundy extensions!

ACCESSORIZING YOUR LOOK

Consider the color choice for your accessories carefully. Pale shoes against your darker skin tones will not work, instead choose vibrant colors to bring energy to your look. In cooler climates, burgundies and purples are great colors; in warmer climates cornflower, blue-green, raspberry, or blue-red are great alternatives to the basic black or white.

YOUR MAKEUP

Many more international cosmetic companies are now catering for the very wide range of different skin colors. You will need to experiment and try a selection of foundations and concealers to find the one that flatters your skin tone. Avoid wearing any shades that look orangey against your skin.

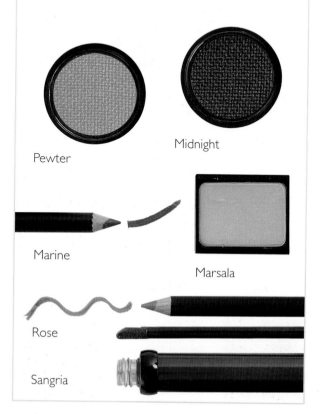

Pewter

Midnight

Marine

Marsala

Rose

Sangria

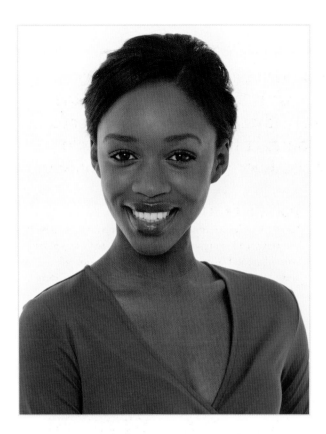

YOUR COLOR COMBINATIONS

These color combinations can be used as block colors or in a print.

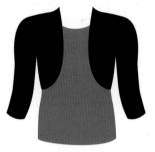

Black & Fuschia

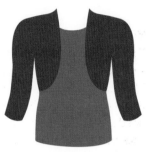

Royal Blue & Cornflower

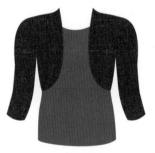

Charcoal & Plum

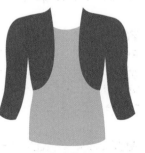

Dark Teal & Light Aqua

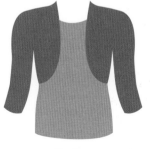

Raspberry & Hot Pink

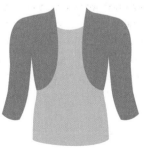

Blue-Green & Duck Egg

YOUR ADDITIONAL COLORS

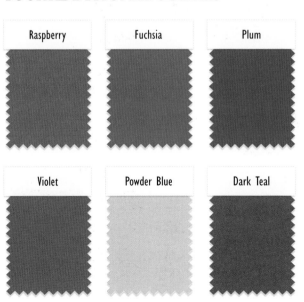

Raspberry	Fuchsia	Plum

Violet	Powder Blue	Dark Teal

ARE YOU A CLEAR ?

DO YOU HAVE ...

- Dark hair?
- Bright eyes that are your most striking feature, be they blue, green, or topaz? If you are dark-skinned there will be noticeable contrast between the white of your eyes and the color of the iris.
- Dark eyebrows and eyelashes?
- Skin that can be any tone from light to dark brown?

YOUR LOOK IS

- Fresh and clear.
- The undertone of your skin may be either warm or cool.
- Your overall look is contrasting between light and dark.
- You have a decidedly clear look.

YOUR IDEAL COLORS

For a master color palette: go to pages 94–95.

HOW TO WEAR YOUR COLORS

Because your look is contrasting (for example, dark hair, bright eyes and for fairer people, porcelain skin), you need to wear your colors in a way that balances this. You will always look good in a contrast of light and dark colors. If you wear sludgy colors like taupe and pewter, liven them up with the brightest shades from your palette. If you dress in a single color, make sure it is one of the most vivid from your palette. If your personality type is one that makes you uncomfortable wearing very bright colors, use accessories to add colors to your look: bright scarves, necklaces, or earrings will also give you the contrast you need.

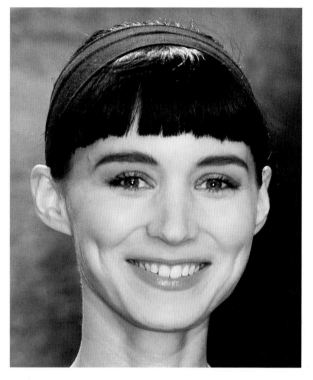

Rooney Mara has typical clear coloring with very bright green eyes, porcelain skin tone, deep eyebrows, and dark hair.

BE AWARE

Basic neutrals like black, charcoal, and black-brown are great staples in your wardrobe, but do wear them with the lighter shades from your palette. You may be tempted to wear white in summer, but combine it with a bright color like scarlet, or even black, to keep a light and dark contrast.

BEING CLEAR

If you are always being complimented on your eyes, you are probably a Clear. Whatever your skin color, you will have a very clear color to the iris of your eye, while the whites will be very bright. Your hair color will have some depth to it, be it dark brown or black. Keep it that way and do not be tempted to go blonde or add highlights.

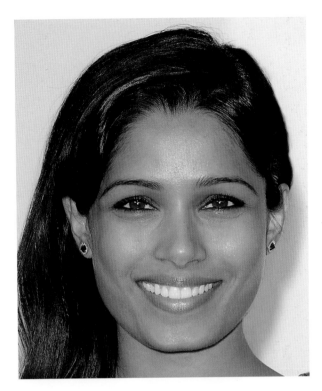

Freida Pinto has stunning, almost jewel-like clear brown eyes, warm olive skin tone, and dark brown hair.

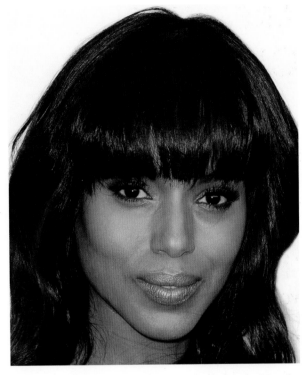

Kerry Washington has amazing contrast between the white and iris of her eyes, which give her a wonderful clear characteristic.

Lowlights and various blends of deep colors may be added if you start to see natural highlights coming. If you go lighter you will no longer be Clear.

TIPS FOR WEARING YOUR COLORS

If you have some warm tones to your eye color and in your hair, try some of the warmer brighter colors from your palette. If your skin is porcelain or has a blue tinge, your may prefer some cooler tones. Whatever you decide, always wear something bright or contrasting. Don't forget that a stunning smile will always enhance your clear look, so regular visits to the dentist shouldn't be overlooked. If you wear glasses, make sure the lenses are nonreflecting so your striking eye color remains visible.

COLORING YOUR HAIR

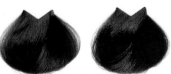

Dark brown   Deep dark brown   Black

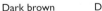

You have the choice of adding wonderful lowlights to your hair color, but also don't forget to condition regularly to keep its shine and luster.

CLEAR COLOR PALETTE

INVESTMENT COLORS

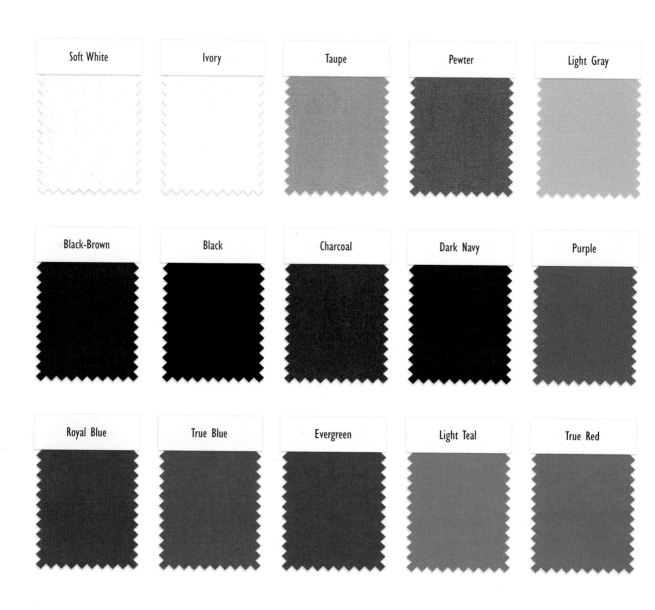

Soft White   Ivory   Taupe   Pewter   Light Gray

Black-Brown   Black   Charcoal   Dark Navy   Purple

Royal Blue   True Blue   Evergreen   Light Teal   True Red

FASHION COLORS

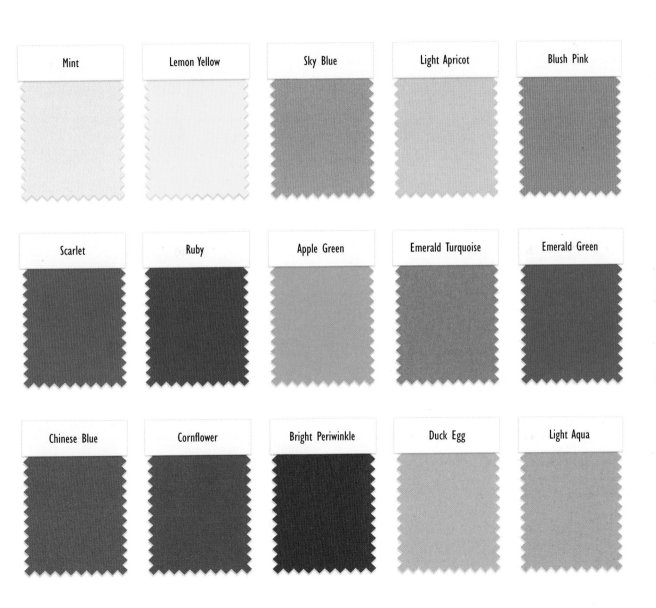

Mint

Lemon Yellow

Sky Blue

Light Apricot

Blush Pink

Scarlet

Ruby

Apple Green

Emerald Turquoise

Emerald Green

Chinese Blue

Cornflower

Bright Periwinkle

Duck Egg

Light Aqua

CLEAR 1

Our first type of Clear has a skin that is porcelain in tone with dark brown eyebrows to frame jewel-like eyes. The contrast between the depth of coloring in the hair, the light skin tone and those brilliant and sparkly eyes make this a very striking look. You will always be someone who is complimented on your fantastically bright eye color.

YOUR COLORS

Your colors are most exciting when worn in contrast, for example ivory with red or charcoal with blush pink. Keep away from smudgy and muted tones or tonal looks. You need to reflect the high contrast of your hair and skin tone with that of your wardrobe. If wearing just one color it needs to be bright and clear such as Chinese blue, bright periwinkle, or apple green. Black is in your palette but it needs to be brought to life either with sparkling jewelry (imagine that little black dress, those jewels, and your eyes sparkling). For formal wear, black needs to be lifted with a pale color such as ivory, lemon yellow, or light peach.

YOUR HAIR

You need to keep the dark tones to your hair—do not be tempted to highlight your hair unless you want to change your dominant coloring type. Lowlights can be flattering on Clears whether warm or cool.

ACCESSORIZING YOUR LOOK

Sparkle, sparkle, sparkle should sum up your attitude to your accessories, whether it is your jewelry, your glasses, your shoes, or even your laptop or tablet cover!

YOUR MAKEUP

To frame your eyes, eyeliners are an essential part of your makeup routine. Use a complementary color to your eyes rather than distracting from them with an unrelated shade. If focusing on your eyes, keep your lip color more subtle using a lip gloss rather than a cream lipstick.

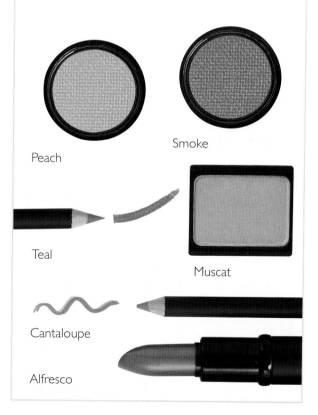

Peach

Smoke

Teal

Muscat

Cantaloupe

Alfresco

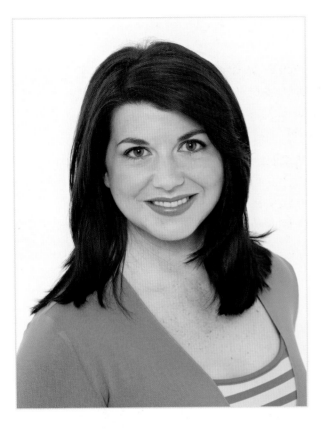

YOUR COLOR COMBINATIONS

These color combinations can be used as block colors or in a print.

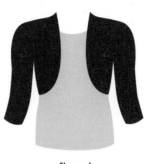

Charcoal
& Peach

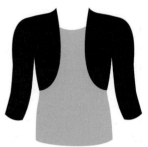

Dark Navy &
Apple Green

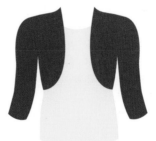

Evergreen &
Lemon Yellow

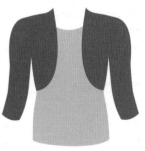

Ruby &
Light Gray

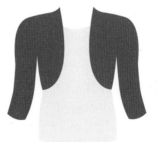

Purple
& Mint

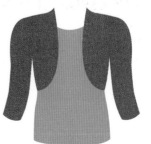

Pewter &
Blush Pink

YOUR ADDITIONAL COLORS

Buttermilk	Light Peach	Peach

Light Gold	Yellow-Green	Light Moss

CLEAR 2

You may be our second type of Clear if you have a medium-depth skin tone with dark hair and striking eyes. There will be a sharpness to your look, which will be wonderfully complemented, as you mature, with the clear tones of your palette both for clothes and makeup. Your fantastically bright eye color will always be noticed and complimented.

YOUR COLORS

Yes, you can wear black, but there are so many other shades that will be interesting on you. Purple is a color that has become increasingly fashionable over the last decade and can be found in the stores all year round. Do not ignore the brighter colors from your palette for outerwear such as apple green or blush pink for a raincoat on a wet dull day. In colder climes go for a bright royal blue, red, or emerald turquoise coat. If wearing your grays and navies, choose a fabric with some sheen such as silk, taffeta, or satin.

YOUR HAIR

If you want to add color to your hair, why not use varying shades of lowlights: two or three shades together will enhance your natural color. Cover any natural highlights with a warm tint, such as gold or copper, which will give the appearance of lowlights. Semi-permanent tints will have the same effect.

ACCESSORIZING YOUR LOOK

Be bold with your accessories. A simple way to add contrast to your look is to use a stunning pashmina in the brightest color imaginable. If you have a defined waist (see page 120) use belts to bring a splash of color to one of your neutrals.

YOUR MAKEUP

For the more mature Clear woman who may not want to wear too much eye makeup, balancing your contrasting look can easily be achieved by using a brighter lipstick. After the last application of lipstick use your lip pencil on the outer edge of your lips to give a firm edge and definition.

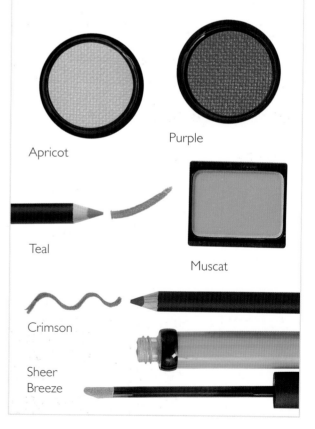

Apricot

Purple

Teal

Muscat

Crimson

Sheer Breeze

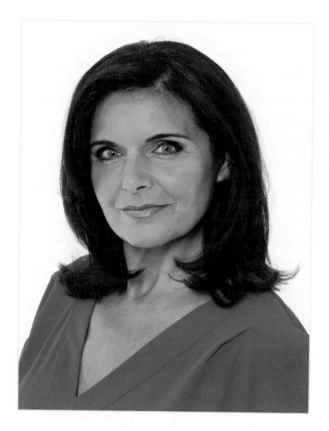

YOUR COLOR COMBINATIONS

These color combinations can be used as block colors or in a print.

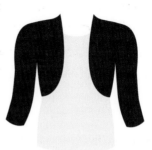

Black-Brown
& Mint

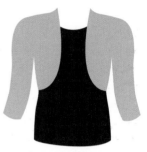

Light Aqua
& Dark Navy

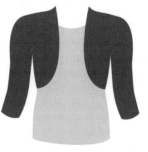

Royal Blue &
Clear Salmon

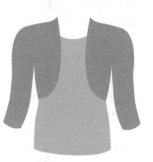

Emerald Turquoise
& Apple Green

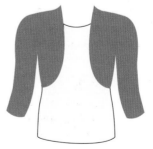

Watermelon
& Ivory

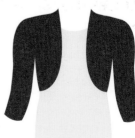

Charcoal
& Lemon

YOUR ADDITIONAL COLORS

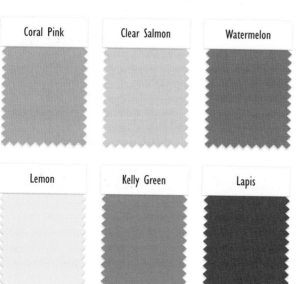

Coral Pink	Clear Salmon	Watermelon

Lemon	Kelly Green	Lapis

CLEAR 3

Our third type of Clear has lots of contrast. You fit this category if the vibrant white of your eyes contrasts against the color of your iris, you have black hair and a brilliant white smile. Your look is dramatic and will call for drama in the color combinations you choose to wear. Don't forget to reflect that clarity and brightness when you choose makeup colors.

YOUR COLORS

You need to think drama when putting colors together. Blacks and reds are the obvious choices, however charcoal may be used with fuchsia, raspberry, and blush pink shades. Adding a contrasting colored jacket to your basic navy pants or skirts is a fun way of introducing variety in your wardrobe. If you happen to want to wear the lighter neutrals from your palette such as taupe and pewter, remember to add a vibrant shade of purple or red with these. Ivory and soft white are in your palette and if worn head to toe need to be put together with a stunning piece of jewelry or perhaps a bright scarf.

YOUR HAIR

Depending on the texture of your hair you may like to leave it natural or you might like to consider changing your look completely with wigs or hair extensions; make sure that you keep to a beautiful shade of dark brown or black. If you change your hair color dramatically, you will no longer be a Clear.

ACCESSORIZING YOUR LOOK

Drama is called for here again and there is no easier way to do it than with accessories. Make sure they are colorful, bold, and make a statement. Check out our advice on pages 138–139 for scale.

YOUR MAKEUP

The boldness and drama of your look also need to be represented in your makeup. Sheen and glitter in your eye makeup will be wonderfully complementary to your look but are best avoided if there are any crinkles in this area. If you have full lips, tone down the shade of your lipstick a little.

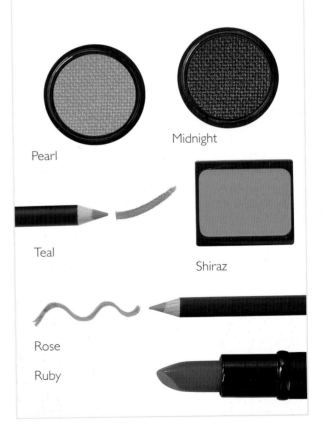

Pearl

Midnight

Teal

Shiraz

Rose

Ruby

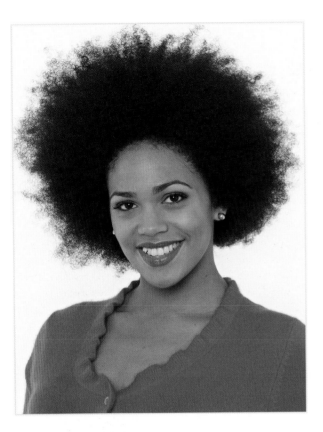

YOUR COLOR COMBINATIONS

These color combinations can be used as block colors or in a print.

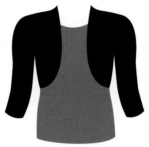

Black &
Fuschia

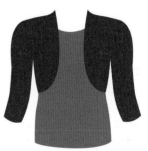

Charcoal
& Violet

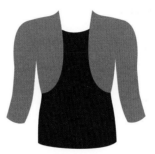

Chinese Blue
& Black-Brown

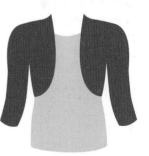

Bright Periwinkle
& Powder Blue

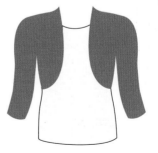

Scarlet &
Soft White

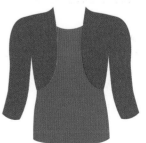

Dark Teal &
Raspberry

YOUR ADDITIONAL COLORS

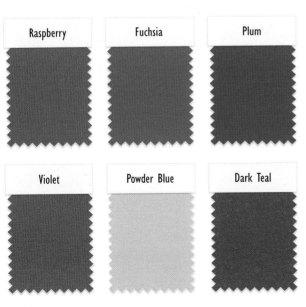

Raspberry	Fuchsia	Plum

Violet	Powder Blue	Dark Teal

ARE YOU A SOFT ?

DO YOU HAVE ...
- Dark blonde (mousey) or light brown hair?
- Eyes that are a soft and muted color, whether blue, brown, hazel, or green, and that often change color?
- Light to dark eyebrows and eyelashes?
- Little contrast between the color of your hair, your eyes, and your skin, which may be any tone from light to dark brown?

YOUR LOOK IS
- Soft, with coloring characteristics that are apparently unrelated and may be confusing. You may have found a little of yourself in each of the previous five dominant coloring types, but you do not fit any of them exactly.
- The undertone of your skin may be either warm or cool.
- The overall depth of your coloring is medium.
- Your look is decidedly soft.

YOUR IDEAL COLORS
For a master color palette: go to pages 104–105.

HOW TO WEAR YOUR COLORS
Because your look is blended, your colors need to be worn "tone-on-tone," with little contrast. You will always look best in tones of medium depth.

A monochromatic look suits you very well. If you wear the darker shades in your palette, balance them with colors that are only one or two tones lighter and avoid high contrast.

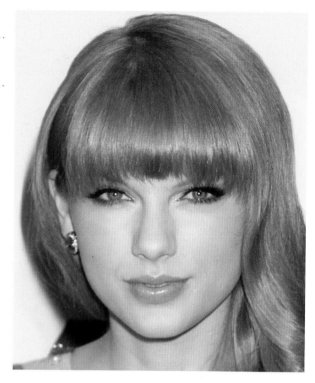

Taylor Swift has dark blonde hair, blended bluey green eyes and an ivory skin tone giving an overall soft look.

BE AWARE
If you like to wear strong, bright colors, choose instead interesting combinations like sapphire and mint, purple and geranium, or damson plum and blush pink. Wear pale shades like soft white or shell with medium-depth colors rather than dark shades.

BEING SOFT
Softs have a blended medium-depth look. The hair may be medium to dark blonde, often highlighted or a light brown. Some women, who were Deeps and are coloring their hair to cover gray, will become Softs. Others might just like to be creative with their image and go from natural dark hair to blonde to have a changeable look. The eye color is often blended, and

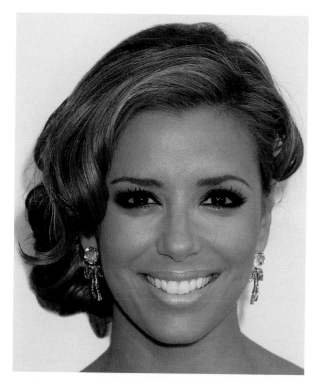

Eva Longoria has stunning dark blonde hair that complements her dark brown eyes and Mediterranean look.

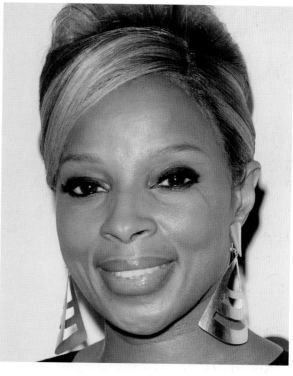

Mary J. Blige loves to play with her hair color so the resulting look is of medium depth and little contrast.

is apt to change color with what they are wearing or even according to mood.

TIPS FOR WEARING YOUR COLORS

The Soft palette is a tonal look but if you are a Creative or a Dramatic you might like to use the soft colors only in contrast and fun color combinations. Black worn near your face is not a complimentary look. If you have green or brown eyes, try some warmer shades; blue eyes are slightly better in cooler tones. Some of you may be neutral in your coloring, in which case you may wear both. Take care with your accessories choices. Softer textures will work better for you, for example suede in preference to leather and matte jewelry rather than very shiny pieces.

COLORING YOUR HAIR

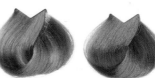
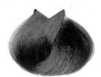

Dark blonde   Light brown   Brown

Softs normally love to play with their hair color but try not to go more than one or two shades lighter or darker than your natural tone.

SOFT COLOR PALETTE

INVESTMENT COLORS

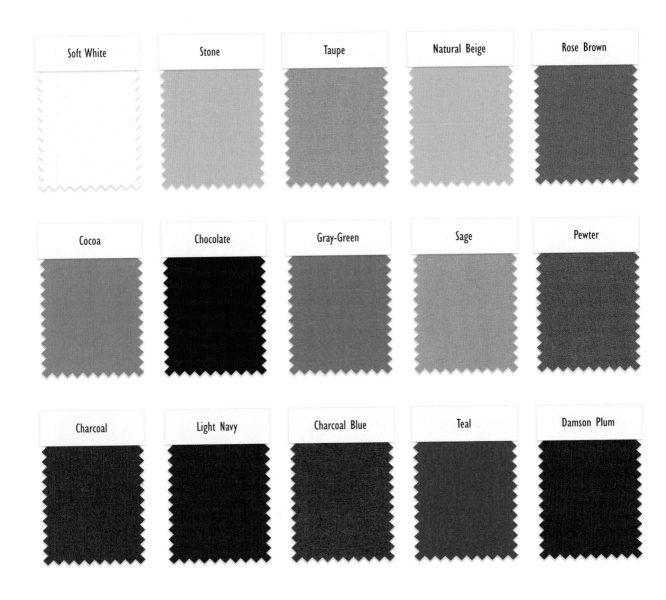

Soft White	Stone	Taupe	Natural Beige	Rose Brown
Cocoa	Chocolate	Gray-Green	Sage	Pewter
Charcoal	Light Navy	Charcoal Blue	Teal	Damson Plum

FASHION COLORS

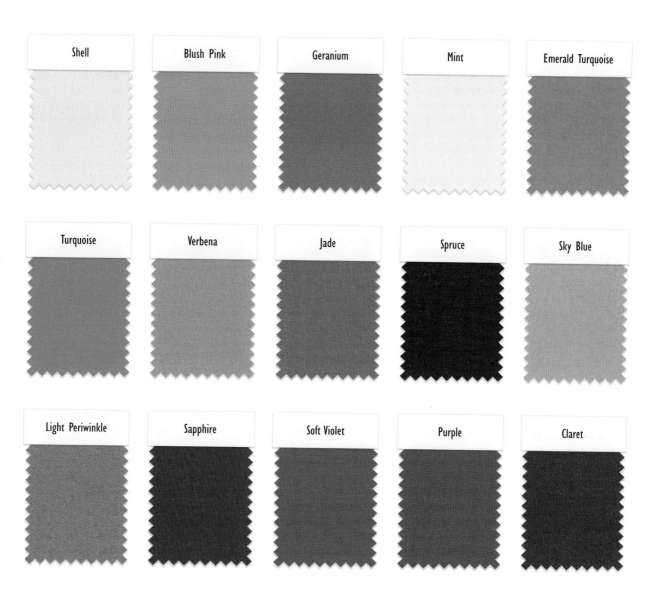

| Shell | Blush Pink | Geranium | Mint | Emerald Turquoise |

| Turquoise | Verbena | Jade | Spruce | Sky Blue |

| Light Periwinkle | Sapphire | Soft Violet | Purple | Claret |

SOFT 1

The first type of Soft has highlighted brown hair, a mid-tone complexion, and soft muted eyes, creating a wonderful blended appearance. Softs are often born blonde and as they get older their hair darkens to a dark mousey blonde that comes to life again once it is highlighted. Remember, highlights are lower maintenance than an all-over tint and look more natural.

YOUR COLORS

To create harmony and balance with your soft blended appearance you will need to wear colors that are tonal (tone-on-tone), for example charcoal blue with sky blue or jade with turquoise. Your other option is to wear your colors within a medium-contrast spectrum: for example pewter with sage or charcoal with verbena. Black worn near the face will not be doing you any favors, however charcoal will work perfectly as an alternative. If the occasion calls for you to wear black, it needs to be in a soft textured fabric such as wool, which absorbs the light so muting the color.

YOUR HAIR

When highlighting your hair, a combination of highlights and lowlights will work best for you, rather than an all-over tint, because this will not look natural. As you mature, continue with the highlights and lowlights to guarantee that youthful head of hair.

ACCESSORIZING YOUR LOOK

When choosing your accessories, think subtle, blended, understated rather than bold and over the top. Metals should be matte rather than shiny. Beads and semiprecious stones should be in natural colors. But, you will be pleased to hear, diamonds are allowed!

YOUR MAKEUP

Your makeup colors are medium depth and you should aim to create an overall blended look. Whatever your lifestyle, do not step out of your home without first applying a little lipstick to put some color on your face—your unmade-up blended look could make you appear tired.

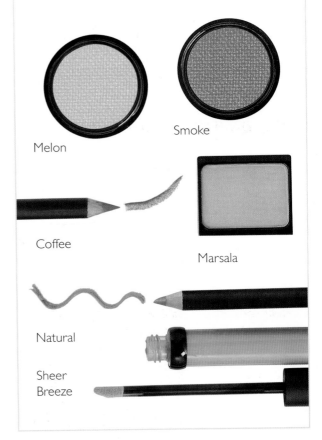

Melon

Smoke

Coffee

Marsala

Natural

Sheer
Breeze

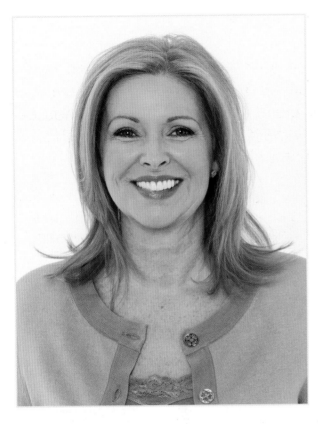

YOUR COLOR COMBINATIONS

These color combinations can be used as block colors or in a print.

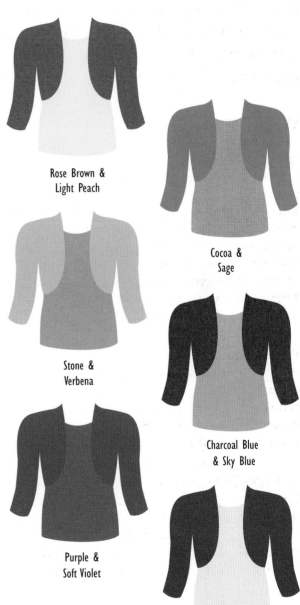

Rose Brown &
Light Peach

Cocoa &
Sage

Stone &
Verbena

Charcoal Blue
& Sky Blue

Purple &
Soft Violet

Claret
& Shell

YOUR ADDITIONAL COLORS

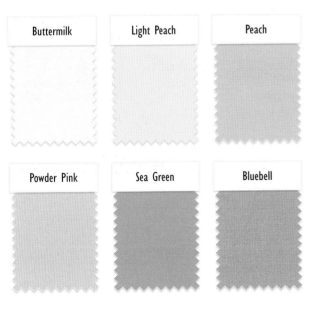

Buttermilk	Light Peach	Peach

Powder Pink	Sea Green	Bluebell

SOFT 2

You fall into our second category of Soft if you were a Deep in your younger days but have developed natural highlights as you have matured. You may choose to lighten the color of your hair to a dark blonde, which will have the effect of softening and lightening your appearance and therefore changing your color palette to Soft.

YOUR COLORS

Women who change palette from Deep to Soft will still need to keep some depth of coloring in their look. The lighter shades in this palette might be used for lingerie, tanks, or as an accent color but not as an overall head-to-toe look. You look wonderful wearing a deep tonal look, such as chocolate with coffee brown and cocoa. Blended patterns such as animal print, are a winner for you. Don't be shy to try red (claret, geranium, or even tomato red) for energy and impact. Wear a textured fabric to soften your appearance.

YOUR HAIR

As you will be probably color-treating your hair, it is essential that you condition it on a regular basis and keep it trimmed to avoid the appearance of over-treated split ends. Your highlights need to be warm and golden rather than ash, which will be aging.

ACCESSORIZING YOUR LOOK

In colder climates, have fun with fake-fur collars and cuffs to add glamour to any outfit. Shawls with texture—knits or anything in mohair—as well as crushed fabrics and fringes work well to soften the look and keep you warm. Experiment and be creative with natural materials like wood, raffia, and leather.

YOUR MAKEUP

Your eyebrows are an essential part of your look so ensure you keep some definition there. Brown-black mascara is more flattering than plain black. Don't forget your eyeliner either in brown or granite. You may need to lighten your lipstick to a medium depth to soften the overall makeup look.

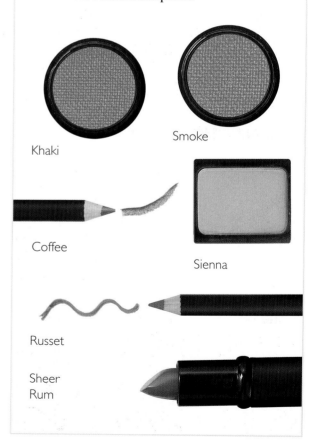

Khaki

Smoke

Coffee

Sienna

Russet

Sheer
Rum

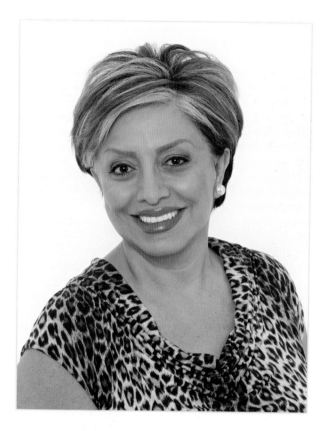

YOUR COLOR COMBINATIONS

These color combinations can be used as block colors or in a print.

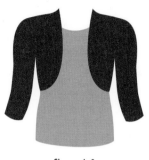

Charcoal & Mustard

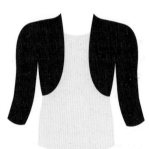

Chocolate & Shell

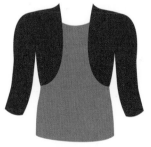

Spruce & Jade

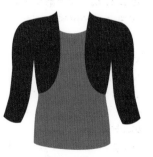

Damson Plum & Soft Violet

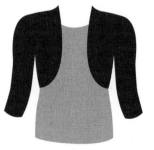

Light Navy & Taupe

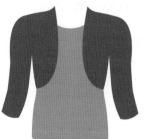

Tomato Red & Pumpkin

YOUR ADDITIONAL COLORS

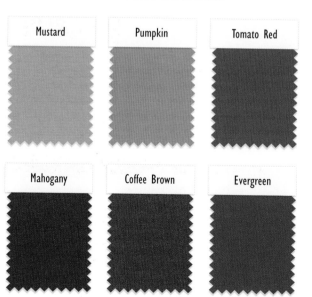

Mustard	Pumpkin	Tomato Red
Mahogany	Coffee Brown	Evergreen

SOFT 3

Unrelated characteristics such as dark brown skin and light hair will make you our third type of Soft. If you are a Deep or Clear and change your hair color, either by tinting your hair or wearing wigs or hair extensions, you may find that your coloring will change too. Just make sure that your clothes and makeup work with your new Soft look.

YOUR COLORS

Because of your darker skin and lighter hair, you will need to soften your look by wearing the darker shades of your palette in tone with the medium-depth shades, such as spruce with teal. Charcoal with pewter would also be a winning combination. Depending on your style personality you may wish to add a splash of color to these combinations, maybe with geranium, blush pink, or turquoise. The lighter shades of your palette, such as shell, natural beige, and stone are great in combination with deeper shades in a pattern. In warmer climates, be careful of wearing light shades from head to toe.

YOUR HAIR

There are many ways to change the look of your hair without having to resort to strong chemical processes. Wigs are the obvious alternative not only to change your color but also the style of your hair. Many women end up with a cabinet full of wigs that they can wear depending on the occasion. If you change the color of your hair regularly, then you may have to change your palette accordingly, and create a new, separate wardrobe.

ACCESSORIZING YOUR LOOK

You may love to go bare-legged; if so make sure your legs are toned and unblemished. If the occasion calls for tights, choose a shade that matches your skin tone.

YOUR MAKEUP

If you have good skin you may simply want to go for a natural look without foundation but do not forget your moisturizer with sun protection. If you do wear makeup, focus on your eyes and do not forget your blush. A cream blush is a good alternative to a powder one when applied directly to the skin.

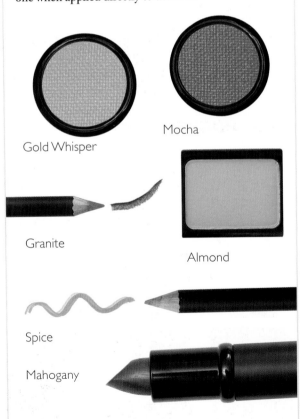

Gold Whisper

Mocha

Granite

Almond

Spice

Mahogany

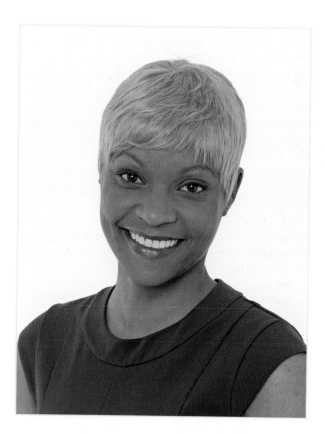

YOUR ADDITIONAL COLORS

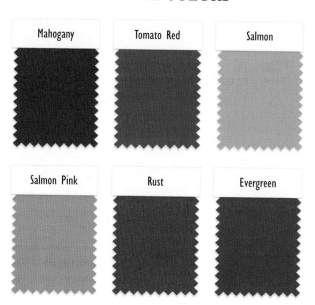

Mahogany	Tomato Red	Salmon

Salmon Pink	Rust	Evergreen

YOUR COLOR COMBINATIONS

These color combinations can be used as block colors or in a print.

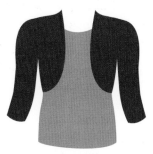

Mahogany &
Salmon Pink

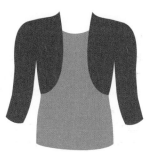

Teal &
Emerald Turquoise

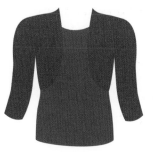

Rust &
Tomato Red

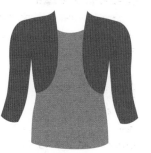

Purple &
Light Periwinkle

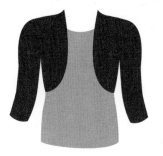

Charcoal
& Sage

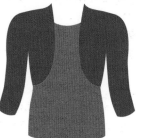

Evergreen &
Rose Brown

COLORS EVERYONE CAN WEAR

There are shades of color within the color spectrum that we refer to as universal colors. This means that they are suitable for all the color types to wear, though they may be worn in different ways. These are great colors to choose for your investment buys and for workwear.

WHAT IS A UNIVERSAL COLOR?

A universal color is one that is of medium depth, neither light nor dark; neutral in undertone, neither warm nor cool; and neutral in clarity, neither clear nor soft. Universal colors are suitable to be worn by everyone, but each coloring type will wear them in a different way, within the guidelines of their palette.

Some of the universal colors, such as stone, taupe, and pewter, are great accessory colors for shoes, handbags, and belts for all coloring types. Turquoise, emerald, and teal are good investment buys for casual and vacation wear as they never go out of fashion. Periwinkle and purple are winners all year round. Mint will lift any darker neutral. True red is a great pick-me-up and accessory color especially if you are shy of wearing it in a garment. Blush pink will add a hint of femininity to any outfit.

EVERYBODY CAN WEAR ANY COLOR

Yes, it is true: everyone *can* wear every color. It is just a matter of understanding the depth, clarity, and tone of the color and relating it to your dominant type. Refer to the page opposite to see how the different dominant types can wear shades of the same color, be it from pastel shades to even black.

UNIVERSAL COLORS

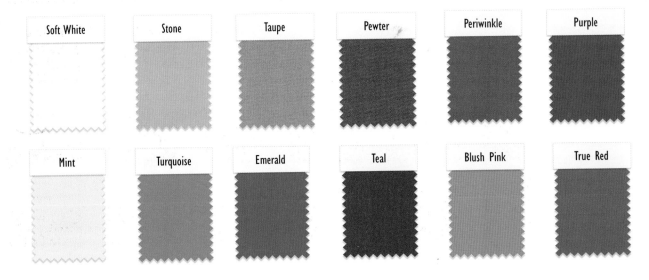

Soft White | Stone | Taupe | Pewter | Periwinkle | Purple

Mint | Turquoise | Emerald | Teal | Blush Pink | True Red

WEARING THE RIGHT SHADE

	LIGHT	DEEP	WARM	COOL	CLEAR	SOFT
PASTELS	Light Apricot	Primrose	Apricot	Icy Violet	Sky Blue	Mint
BLUES	Sky Blue	True Blue	Light Periwinkle	Cornflower	Chinese Blue	Sapphire
GREENS	Apple Green	Forest Green	Moss	Blue-Green	Evergreen	Verbena
AQUAS	Light Aqua	Teal	Turquoise	Peppermint	Light Teal	Jade
PURPLES	Violet	Royal Purple	Purple	Light Periwinkle	Bright Periwinkle	Soft Violet
PINKS	Pastel Pink	Blush Pink	Coral	Rose Pink	Hot Pink	Blush Pink
REDS	Geranium	True Red	Orange-Red	Blue-Red	Scarlet	Claret
BLACKS & GRAYS	Light Gray	Black	Gray-Green	Medium Gray	Charcoal	Pewter

HOW TO WEAR BLACK

Black has probably become the basic color in most women's closets and is readily available all year round, in all styles and at all price categories. It is often the first choice for evening wear—the classic little black dress (LBD)—and many women use black as a staple "uniform" for their working wardrobe.

It is commonly believed that black is slimming. This is, however, only true if it is worn in the correct style and fabric. As we have seen earlier in this chapter, there are many alternatives to black in everyone's palette, be they chocolate, charcoal, or navy, to make them look appropriate for work or formal occasions, and slimmer, too. We believe that it is not the color you wear but how you wear it that makes it a success.

THE KEY TO SUCCESS

Everyone can still have their LBD depending on the fabric it is made from, how much flesh is on show and what accessories and makeup are worn.

ALL SHADES OF BLACK

Texture and weave will alter the way in which the light is absorbed by the fabric. The appearance of black will soften when you use a textured fabric; this is a great way for Softs and Lights to introduce black into their wardrobe. All types of knits, both synthetic and pure wool, will soften black, as well as tweeds. Sheer fabrics also "lighten" black and shiny fabrics, such as silk or satin, will sparkle and reflect the light.

SHOWING FLESH

Very few women—except the Deeps—will be able to wear a black roll-neck sweater. Indeed, a Deep is the only coloring type that can wear a dark color on its own near the face. To help wear black successfully, leave enough flesh on show with a lower or open neckline.

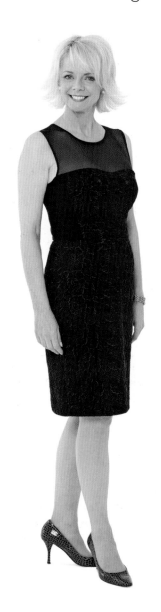

ACCESSORIZE YOUR BLACK WITH SCARVES

Scarves are a wonderful addition to any wardrobe and are a foolproof ally to ensure that black works for you whatever your coloring. Choose your scarf in your favorite color(s) and wear it near your face so that the colors reflecting onto your face are in harmony and balance with your natural coloring. There are many ways of wearing scarves, and they will add style depending on what shape they are (pashmina style, large square, oblong) and how you wear them.

ACCESSORIZE YOUR BLACK WITH JEWELRY

Alternatively, wearing jewelry, whether the real McCoy or costume, is a sure-fire way to make your black outfit flattering. The light will reflect on metals and beads, giving a lift and bringing out your natural coloring. Make sure that the colors of the beads are in your palette. Warmer skin tones are best in gold, copper, and bronze; cooler skin tones are best in silver, platinum, and pewter. Diamonds are perfect on everyone!

Makeup

Ensure that you are wearing the right shades of makeup for your color palette. Many women make the mistake of wearing too strong a shade of lipstick or blusher when wearing black, especially in the evening. Also avoid the temptation to be overdramatic with your eyeliner and eye shadow colors.

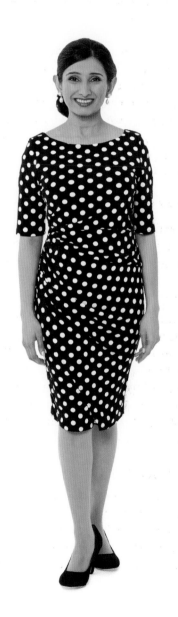

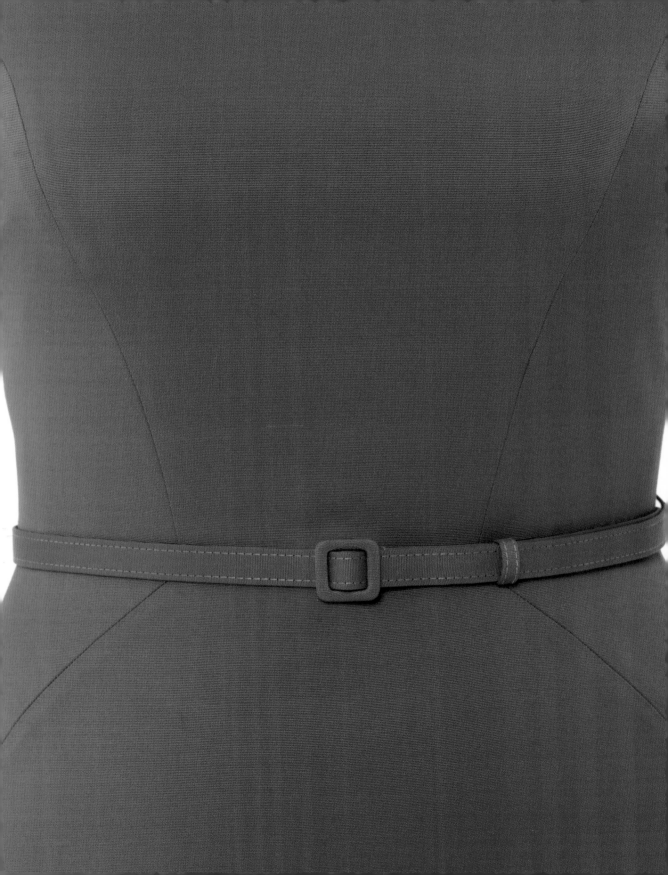

5

SIZE DOESN'T MATTER, SHAPE DOES

WOMEN SHOULD HAVE CURVES

Fashion magazines and the runways may be full of very slim models with a fragile look, but women are actually designed to have curves. It's natural, it's feminine, it's sexy and most men say they prefer curvy women.

When it comes to looking good, it's not your size or shape that matters, it's the fit of your clothes. Wearing the right clothes is not about following the latest fashion or fad, it's about choosing what actually suits you and what makes you feel comfortable and confident.

By knowing your basic body shape and understanding the guidelines for choosing the types of clothes that will accentuate your good features and minimize your less-than-perfect areas, you will be able to dress in the way that suits you best. You will also be able to see how to make subtle changes to the way you put your wardrobe together.

The choice of clothes is so varied that you should always be able to find something that will complement your body shape, scale, proportions, and coloring.

BODY SHAPES

Clothing is either constructed along straight lines, which give a garment a more rigid, structured form, or along curved lines, which give a more fluid shape that tends to follow the curves of the body shape.

You cannot alter your basic body line by diet or exercise. It will remain essentially the same throughout your life because your body line is based on your skeleton as well as your genes. The distribution of body fat is also dependent on your genes. If you have a tendency to carry extra weight on your hips, you will almost certainly have a proportionally smaller waist; conversely, women who carry extra weight around their tummies will have straight hips and bottoms.

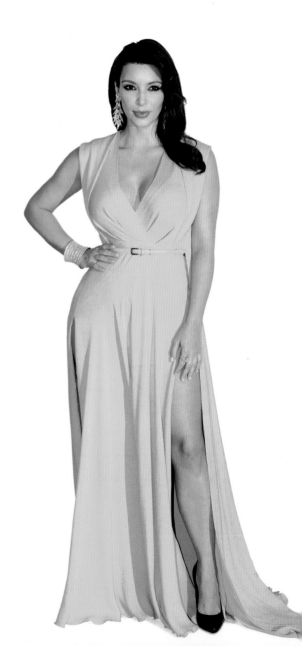

Biologically, women are designed to carry more fat beneath their skin than men (the original hunter-gatherers), and we actually need a few curves in order for our bodies to work efficiently. Fatty deposits around the hips, legs, and arms are normal and should not be viewed as worrying health indicators (unless you feel you are overweight).

When most women stand in front of a mirror, they focus on all the things they would like to change about their bodies. On the following pages you will learn how to recognize your assets and show them off, and how to play down the parts of your body that you are not so happy with. The objective is for you to understand your shape, to be positive about it, and to make the most of what nature has given you.

Whether you are petite or have a fuller figure, the cut of the clothes that will flatter you the best will depend on your basic body shape. For example, if you have a Full Hourglass figure, wearing softer lines is recommended. The only difference between what suits a petite or fuller-figured woman of this body shape will be the size of the pattern and the weight of the fabric in which the garment is made.

The pictures on either side demonstrate how the most shapely of women can look marvelous as long as she chooses the right fabric, in the right cut. It is a matter of understanding what suits you—remember size doesn't matter, shape does!

THE ILLUSION OF A BALANCED BODY

When choosing clothes, your aim is to create the illusion of having a balanced body, a Neat Hourglass figure with:
• Shoulders and hips in line
• A defined bust
• A waist, even with a softly curved tummy
• A curved bottom
• Perfect proportions

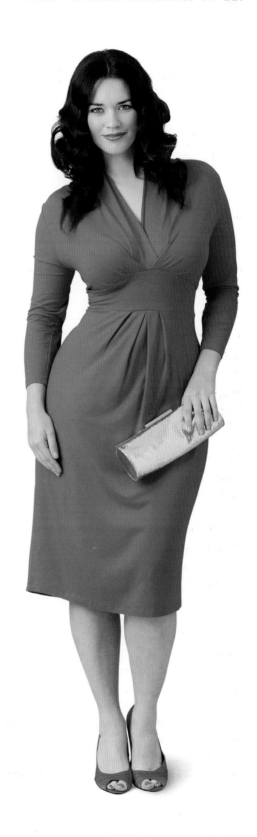

WHAT BODY SHAPE ARE YOU ?

If you want to look slimmer and feel more confident when buying clothes, then it is crucial to consider how to dress all the individual parts of your body, rather than your entire body all at once.

ARE YOU STRAIGHT OR CURVY?

Although understanding your basic body shape is still important, working out whether your body is straight and angular or round and curvy will point you in the right direction for choosing clothing to make you look slimmer. It could also be that your upper body is straighter than your curvy lower half, or vice versa. The charts on the right will help you to decide what overall shape your body is.

Look at the chart on the right while you stand in front of a mirror in clothes that show your shape off. Look at your shoulders: are they straight across or do they slope down? Stand sideways, still looking into the mirror: is the side view like the silhouette of our model in red? If so you have a straight back and flat bottom; or are you more like our model in the brown dress with a curved back and curvy bottom?

Once you have determined which bits of you are straighter or curvier, you need to consider the actual construction of your clothes. Straighter bodies need straighter constructions; curvier bodies need softer and more shaped constructions.

If you found that you are a combination, then you might need straight constructions in soft fabrics. Perhaps a crisp cotton above the waist, with a softer fabric below, is the answer for you. Or try a shift dress in a soft cotton jersey.

HOW TO ASSESS YOUR UPPER BODY

	Straight	Curvy
Face	Square, rectangle or oval	Oval or round
Shoulder line	Straight	Straight or curvy
Arms	Straight upper arms	Full upper arms
Bust	Small to average bust	Full bust
Back	Straight	Curved
Midriff/ ribcage	Straight	Curved
Waist	Not defined	Defined

HOW TO ASSESS YOUR LOWER BODY

	Straight	Curvy
Tummy	Full	Full
Bottom	Flattish	Curvy
Hips	Flattish	Curvy
Thighs	Slim	Full
Calves	Straight	Curvy
Ankles	Full	Shapely

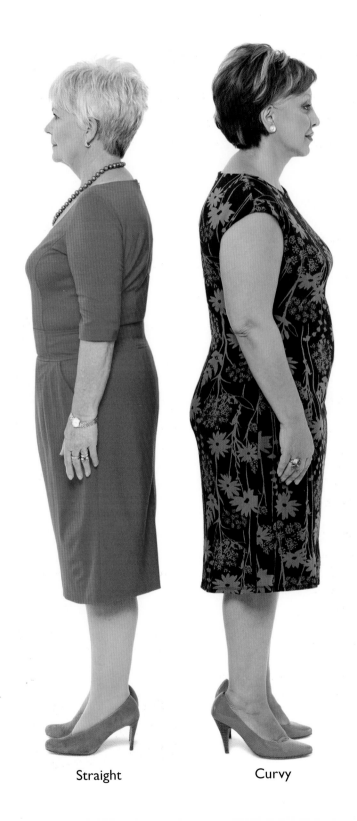

Straight   Curvy

HOW TO IDENTIFY YOUR BODY SHAPE

To identify your basic body shape, read the questions in the boxes below and try to find the one that matches you. If you don't fit exactly into just one shape, choose the one that most closely resembles you. Then turn to the relevant section to discover your clothing guidelines.

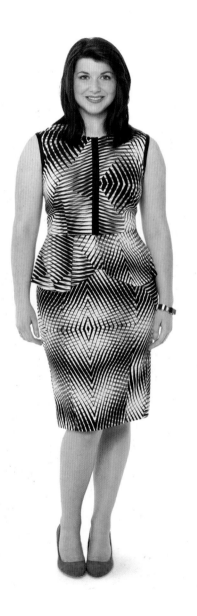

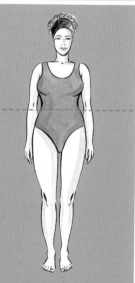

NEAT HOURGLASS

DO YOU

- Wear the same size top and bottom?
- Have a clearly defined waist?
- Have a clearly defined bust?
- Have a curved bottom?

Go to pages 124–125

FULL HOURGLASS

DO YOU

- Buy a slightly larger top for your bust?
- Find that waistbands are often too large?
- Find that a straight skirt rises up?
- Feel comfortable in more fluid fabrics?

Go to pages 126–127

DEFINING YOUR BODY SHAPE

We are not all necessarily made in a perfect mold to fit a recognizable shape. You may be a combination of two different shapes, but this is not an insurmountable problem. Just see where you think you fit in the most, according to the description of each shape. If the description for the top half is one shape, but for the hips and below the waist, you fit another shape, then use the advice for the top half from the right section and for the lower half from the other. If you think you are a Neat Hourglass but still have fit problems, it may be that you have some challenges with scale or proportions—see pages 136–139. Understanding your height, scale, and proportions are just as important as recognizing your shape and sometimes will be the making or breaking of your look.

TRIANGLE ▲	OVAL ●	RECTANGLE ■	INVERTED TRIANGLE ▼
DO YOU	**DO YOU**	**DO YOU**	**DO YOU**
• Wear a larger size on your bottom half than your top?	• Have rounded shoulders?	• Have shoulders and hips in line?	• Have an athletic build?
• Have a clearly defined waist?	• Have fullness in the tummy area?	• Have no waist definition?	• Have wider shoulders than hips?
• Have narrower shoulders than hips?	• Have wonderfully shapely legs?	• Have flat hips and bottom?	• Have a straight ribcage?
• Carry weight on your hips or thighs?	• Feel uncomfortable when clothes are tucked in?	• Carry any extra weight around your middle?	• Prefer an uncluttered look?
Go to pages 128–129	Go to pages 130–131	Go to pages 132–133	Go to pages 134–135

NEAT HOURGLASS

Lucky you! You have a balanced body with your top half in proportion to your bottom half. This means that your clothes don't need to work hard at evening out your shape and can simply follow your natural curves.

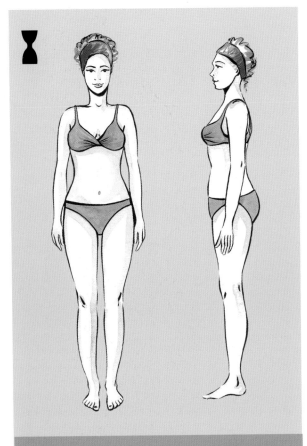

YOUR BUILD IS CHARACTERIZED BY

- A defined bust
- A defined waist
- A neat bottom
- Neat hips

YOUR GOLDEN RULES

- Show off your body by wearing clothes that define your waist, enhance your bust and highlight your hips and bottom.
- Avoid wearing clothes that hide your body line, or you risk looking an extra seven to nine pounds (three to four kilos) heavier than you are.

YOUR CLOTHING LINES

- **Jackets** Fitted, with waist definition.
- **Tops** Shaped, crossovers, or wraps.
- **Skirts** Straight, paneled, flip, bias-cut, soft pleats, or full, preferably with a waistband and some shaping (darts) over the hips and bottom.
- **Pants** Any type, with a waistband (see above).
- **Jeans** Designed for women's bodies.
- **Dresses** Any style, either shaped or belted.
- **Coats** All shapes, as long as they have some shape at the waist or a belt.
- **Swimwear** As long as your proportions are good, you can wear any style (see illustration left).

YOUR BEST FABRICS

Choose fabrics that are light to medium in weight and texture. These will skim the curves of your body:

- Cotton
- Linen
- Silk
- Tightly woven gabardine to relaxed wool crepe
- All cotton jerseys and polyesters
- All knits

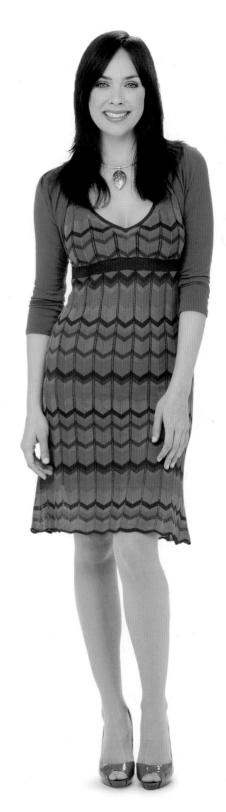

YOUR BEST PATTERNS

Because the top and bottom half of your body are in balance, you are able to wear most types of pattern:

• Stripes
• Abstract
• Checks
• Spots
• Florals
• Paisleys

YOU SHOULD AVOID

• Boxy jackets
• Pants or skirts that have no shaping
• Straight tunics
• Men's shirts
• Baggy sweaters and sportswear
• Too much layering

For more on proportions: go to pages 136–137

For more on scale: go to pages 138–139

For more on who can wear what: go to pages 142–151

For your capsule wardrobe: go to page 172

FULL HOURGLASS

Wow! You have the most feminine body shape with full curves in all the right places. By choosing clothes that are fluid and shaped, you will be able to accentuate your curves rather than cover them up.

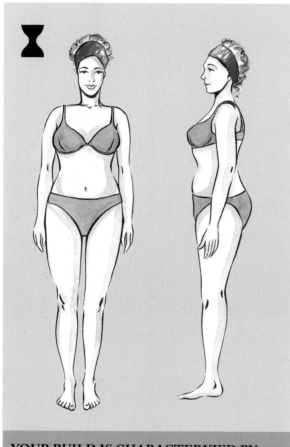

YOUR BUILD IS CHARACTERIZED BY

- A full bust
- A small waist
- A rounded bottom
- Rounded hips

YOUR GOLDEN RULES

- It is important to wear clothes that follow your body line instead of those that are straight and constricting.
- Choose fabrics carefully. Avoid heavy or stiff materials or you'll end up with tops and jackets that are two to three sizes bigger than you need them to be just to accommodate your curves.

YOUR CLOTHING LINES

- **Jackets** Shaped, with shawl collars; waterfall, deconstructed, or cardigan style.
- **Tops** Shaped, crossovers, or wraps, in soft fabrics.
- **Skirts** Flip, bias, or soft pleats, and ideally adjustable at the waist.
- **Pants** Plain with side zippers, cropped, or straight leg.
- **Dresses** Shaped, wrap, bias-cut, tea dress, belted, princess, or puffball.
- **Coats** Shawl collar, single-breasted, or shaped.
- **Swimwear** Underwiring or support is essential. Avoid stripes and detailing at the bust and hips.

YOUR BEST FABRICS

Should be light to medium weight, with little texture. If choosing cotton or linen, look for fabrics cut on the bias to give movement and accommodate your curves:
- Silk and chiffon
- Relaxed wool crepe
- All cotton jerseys and polyesters
- Fine knits
- Fabric that gives and stretches
- Spandex, the best friend of the Full Hourglass

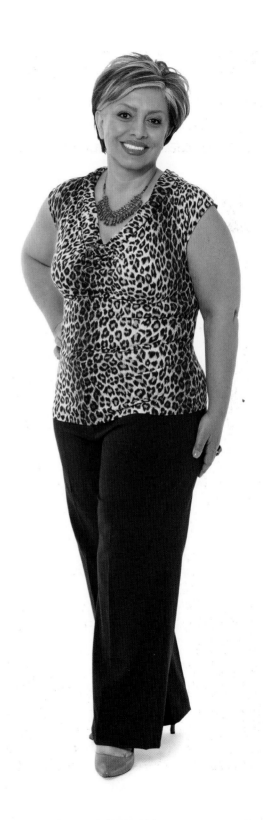

YOUR BEST PATTERNS

Avoid geometric patterns because lines will not lie straight over your curves. Instead, opt for more fluid shapes such as:

- Spots
- Florals
- Paisleys
- Circles and squiggles

YOU SHOULD AVOID

- Classic jeans (too many pockets)
- Straight skirts, except in soft fabrics with some spandex
- Boxy, double-breasted jackets
- Straight tunics
- Front-opening shirts and blouses
- Baggy sweaters and sportswear
- Too much layering
- Crisp fabrics
- Stripes and checks

For more on proportions: go to pages 136–137

For more on scale: go to pages 138–139

For more on who can wear what: go to pages 142–151

For your capsule wardrobe: go to page 173

TRIANGLE

Great! You can bring all the attention to the top half of your body. You are often referred to as pear-shaped, so with your choice of clothes you should aim to accentuate your bust and minimize your bottom and hips.

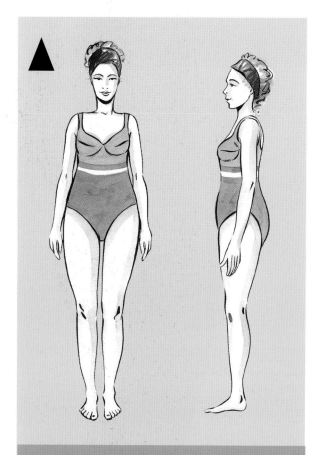

YOUR BUILD IS CHARACTERIZED BY

- Full hips or thighs
- A defined waist
- Shoulders that may slope and are narrower than your hips
- A top half that appears small

YOUR GOLDEN RULES

- Your jackets and tops need to finish either above or below the widest point of your hips and bottom.
- Layering on your top half creates visual interest and draws the eye upward.
- Buy jackets or tops that fit your shoulders rather than your hips—you can always leave the bottom button undone.

YOUR CLOTHING LINES

- **Jackets** Details, collars, pockets, buttons, or double-breasted are excellent.
- **Tops** Patterned, horizontal stripes, twin-sets, vests, T-shirts, and ruffles.
- **Skirts** Simple lines: long flip, bias-cut, or paneled.
- **Pants** Plain with side zipper,s drawstring, or flared (for long legs).
- **Dresses** Separates work better, or wraps.
- **Coats** Square shoulders or wide collars.
- **Swimwear** Keep detailing above the waist. Beware of high-cut styles that finish at your widest point (see illustration left).

YOUR BEST FABRICS

Your aim is to balance out your body shape, so certain fabrics will work best on your lower half:

- Light- to medium-weight fabrics with minimum texture are best
- Soft, fluid fabrics that drape easily, such as wool crepe, cotton jersey, knits, fabrics cut on the bias, silks

Other fabrics that will flatter and draw attention to your top half are:
• Light fabrics worn layered
• Medium- to heavyweight fabrics
• Texture, which adds volume
• Cotton and linen
• All types of woolen fabrics
• Crisper fabrics, which add bulk

YOUR BEST PATTERNS

Any pattern, such as florals and horizontal stripes, is a great way to draw attention to the upper half of your body. Always wear plain colors below the waist.

YOU SHOULD AVOID

• Jeans (too many pockets)
• Straight skirts
• Details on skirts and pants
• Halternecks and raglan sleeves
• Tight-fitting, single-layered tops
• Tops and jackets that finish at your widest point

For more on proportions: go to pages 136–137

For more on scale: go to pages 138–139

For more on who can wear what: go to pages 142–151

For your capsule wardrobe: go to page 174

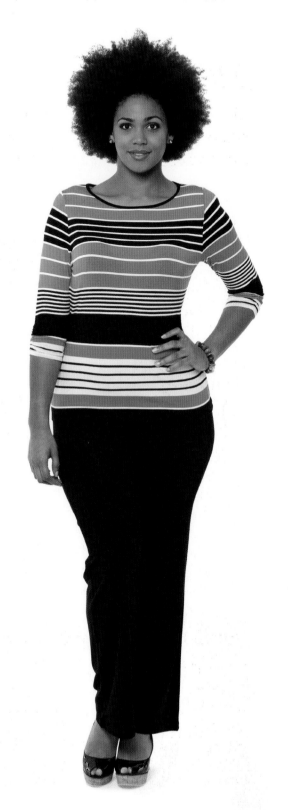

OVAL

Brilliant! Proportionally you have a flat bottom and hips. Your problem area is your central torso, so wherever possible use accessories to draw the eye to the area above your bust and below your hips. Your aim is to give the impression of a slightly longer body.

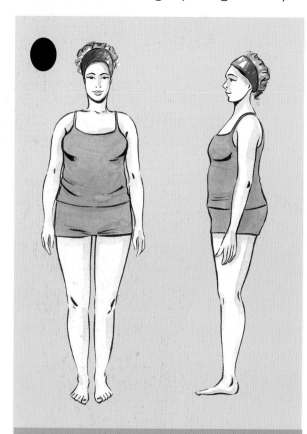

YOUR BUILD IS CHARACTERIZED BY

- Rounded or sloping shoulder line
- Curved back
- Fullness around the middle
- Flattish bottom curving down to the hips and balancing with the shoulders to create an oval

YOUR GOLDEN RULES

- Make sure the clothes that you wear hang from your shoulders.
- Clothing lines need to be straight, and fabrics soft to avoid any unnecessary volume or bulkiness.
- Keep any detail above the bust line and below the hip line.
- Accessorize, accessorize, accessorize.

YOUR CLOTHING LINES

- **Jackets** Cardigan-style, waterfall, or deconstructed.
- **Tops** Simple lines, no details.
- **Skirts** Wrap, flip, or paneled.
- **Pants** Drawstrings, straight, or cropped.
- **Dresses** A-line (trapeze), wrap, drop waistline.
- **Coats** A-line, cardigan-style, big wrap.
- **Swimwear** Try a tankini or tank top that covers the middle and isn't too figure-hugging (see illustration left). For more cover, use a sarong. Details on the shoulders draw the eye toward your face.

YOUR BEST FABRICS

The key is to choose soft, fluid fabrics that hang well and don't cling or hug the figure. Stiff or thick fabric will add unwelcome girth.

- Soft cottons and linens
- Wool crepe
- Cotton jersey
- Knits
- Silks

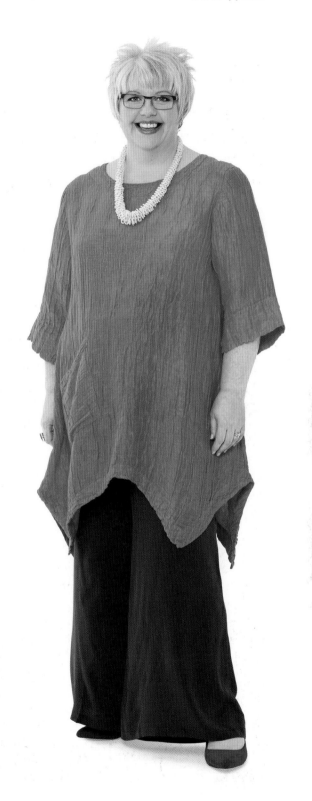

YOUR BEST PATTERNS

Try to go for muted and subtle patterns as much as possible; anything too bold will overpower.
- Soft or faded stripes
- Squiggles and spots
- Abstract florals or paisleys

YOU SHOULD AVOID

- Stiff fabrics
- Pockets
- Gathered waistlines or any other details over the tummy area
- Sharp, angular details such as lapels
- Vibrant and dramatic patterns over the torso
- Small details on your garments, such as small buttons and pockets
- Finishing any garment at the fullest part of your torso

For more on proportions: go to pages 136–137

For more on scale: go to pages 138–139

For more on who can wear what: go to pages 142–151

For your capsule wardrobe: go to page 175

RECTANGLE

Lucky you! You are the one with flat hips and a flat bottom. However, some Rectangles will also have a fuller bust, which gives a softer edge to their shape. Your main aim is to soften those edges even more and create the appearance of curves.

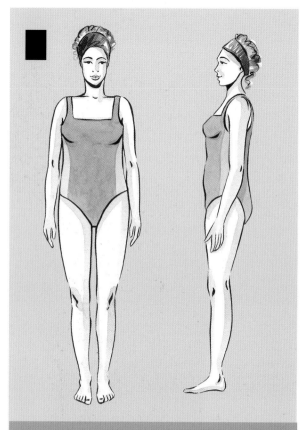

YOUR BUILD IS CHARACTERIZED BY

- Straight shoulder line
- Straight hips and bottom
- Very little waist definition
- Straight ribcage

YOUR GOLDEN RULES

- Use details on your hips and bottom to create shape.
- Avoid details at the waist, such as noticeable waistbands or belts.
- Keep your clothing line straight.
- Go for the uncluttered look.

YOUR CLOTHING LINES

- **Jackets** Structured and shaped.
- **Tops** Simple, clean lines.
- **Skirts** Crossover, straight, paneled, narrow pleats, dropped panel.
- **Pants** The choice is yours.
- **Dresses** Simple, straight lines, or shifts.
- **Coats** Straight lines with some emphasis on the waist.
- **Swimwear** On a one-piece, a central panel in a darker shade gives the illusion of a slimmer shape, as do square necklines (see illustration left). Avoid high-waisted bikini bottoms and choose geometric patterns.

YOUR BEST FABRICS

Most Rectangles can wear crisp fabrics, but if you have a full bust, slightly softer fabrics work better.
- Wool crepe and woven wool
- Cottons and linens
- Cotton jersey and lightweight tweeds
- Fine knits

YOUR BEST PATTERNS

Geometric patterns work best for you because your body is straight.

• Vertical stripes
• Checks
• Geometrics
• Squiggles and spots

YOU SHOULD AVOID

• Frills and flounces
• Gathered waistlines
• Soft, floppy, and fluffy fabrics
• Bias cuts
• Belted jackets and coats
• Florals and paisleys
• Very bulky fabrics, which will hide your shape
• Tucking any garment into a waistband

For more on proportions: go to pages 136–137

For more on scale: go to pages 138–139

For more on who can wear what: go to pages 142–151

For your capsule wardrobe: go to page 176

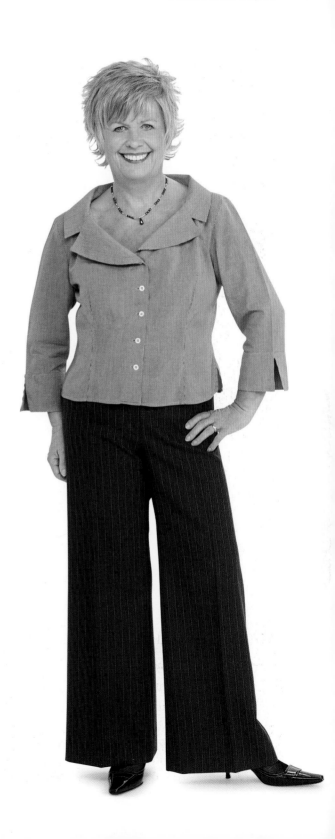

INVERTED TRIANGLE

Magnificent! You have great shoulders—halternecks are made for you.
To balance the upper and lower parts of your body, you need to highlight
your hips and bottom, focusing all attention below your waist.

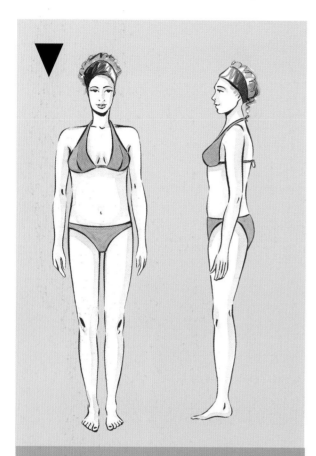

YOUR BUILD IS CHARACTERIZED BY

- Straight and squared shoulder line
- Little definition between waist/hips
- Flat hips and bottom
- A bottom half that seems smaller than your top half

YOUR GOLDEN RULES

- You will need to ensure that there is minimum detail on your shoulder line; keep this area as simple as possible.
- Your clothing line needs to be straight, clean and sharp.
- Your silhouette should be uncluttered.

YOUR CLOTHING LINES

- **Jackets** Constructed, or shaped with angular lines (revered collars).
- **Tops** Simple lines.
- **Skirts** Straight, paneled, A-line, or straight jeans-style.
- **Pants** Any style—pockets and details will accentuate your bottom.
- **Dresses** Simple, straight lines, shifts, or separates.
- **Coats** Straight lines with a slightly shaped waistline and no belt.
- **Swimwear** Halter and square necklines work well, as do details on the hips. Avoid floral patterns. Go for styles where tops and bottoms are sold separately.

YOUR BEST FABRICS

Crisp, constructed fabrics work best for you because your body line is straight and angled.

- Crisp cottons and linens
- Gabardine and fine wool
- Satins and crisp silks
- Ribbed fabrics

YOUR BEST PATTERNS

You can wear patterns above and below the waistline, but they must be geometric to balance the clothing line.

- Stripes
- Checks
- Geometrics
- Squiggles and spots

YOU SHOULD AVOID

- Frills and flounces
- Gathered waistlines
- Tiered skirts
- Epaulettes
- Soft, floppy, and fluffy fabrics
- Bias cuts
- Full circular gathered skirts
- Lightweight sheer fabrics

For more on proportions: go to pages 136–137

For more on scale: go to pages 138–139

For more on who can wear what: go to pages 142–151

For your capsule wardrobe: go to page 177

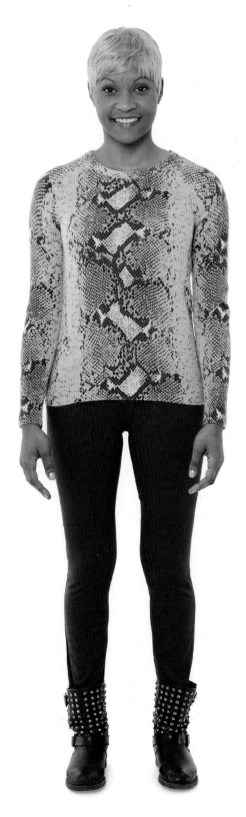

PROPORTIONS

When you look at proportions, you are considering the relationship of your body to your legs, as well as the position of your waist. Once you understand your body proportions, you'll be able to combine clothes that appear to adjust any imbalances and give the illusion of perfect proportions.

THE POSSIBLE COMBINATIONS

- balanced rise + balanced legs = balanced waist
- short rise + long legs = high-waisted
- long rise + average to short legs = high-waisted
- short rise + average to short legs = low-waisted
- long rise + short legs = low-waisted

ASSESSING YOUR PROPORTIONS

Stand in front of a mirror so that you can see your silhouette. Place your hands on your natural waistline. Then place the flat of one hand underneath your bust, and the other below the first hand. If you can easily place two hands widthwise between your bust and waistline, you are low-waisted and may be slightly shorter on the leg. If you have a struggle to get the second hand in, you have long legs and may be high-waisted. If you can get approximately 1½ hands in, you have perfect proportions. You may feel that you have a large bottom, but it could be that you are just long in the rise.

CREATING PERFECT PROPORTIONS

Balanced waist (balanced rise + average legs)

You are lucky in having perfect proportions, with the length of your body and legs in balance with each other. Remember what your height, scale, and body shape are and follow the guidelines given in the appropriate section of this book (pages 118–135) whenever you go clothes shopping. This will ensure that you only buy what suits you the best.

High-waisted (short rise + long legs)

Create the illusion of lowering your waist:
- Dropped waistlines or hipsters.
- Skirts and pants without waistbands.
- Low-slung belts.
- Long jackets and tops.
- Volume or pattern on your legs.
- Long tops and long skirts.
- Don't tuck in tops.

High-waisted (long rise + average to short legs)

Create the illusion of lowering your waist without shortening your legs:
- Low waistlines or hipsters.
- Skirts and pants without waistbands.
- Low-slung belts.
- High heels.
- Long jackets and tops with narrow skirts or pants.
- Don't clutter your leg area.
- Don't tuck in tops.

Low-waisted (short rise + average to short legs)

Create the illusion of raising your waist without shortening your legs:
- Tuck-in or belting.
- Short tops.
- Minimal details in the rise area.
- Short jackets with long or short skirts.
- Shift-style dresses.
- Long jackets with short skirts or narrow pants.
- High heels.
- Don't clutter your leg area.

Low-waisted (long rise + short legs)

Create the illusion of raising your waist and lengthening your legs:

• Tuck-in or belting.
• Short tops and jackets.
• Details such as pockets or trims in the rise area.

• Keep to one color from waist to toe.
• High heels.
• Shift-style dresses.
• Don't clutter your leg area.

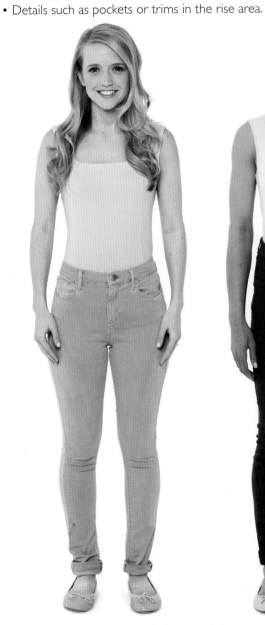

Low waist

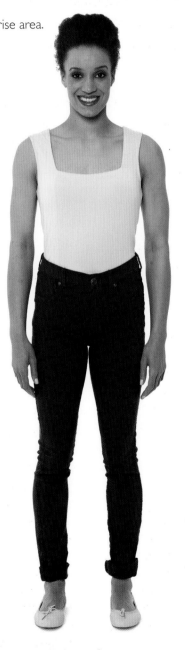

Balanced waist

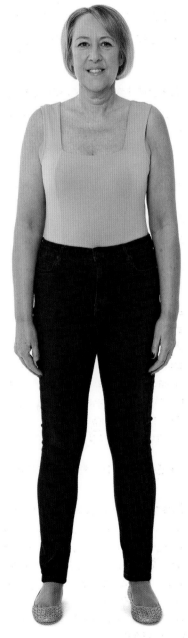

High waist

SCALE

Scale is a combination of height and bone structure. Your scale may be petite, average, or grand, and will determine the size of patterns, the weight of fabrics and how much texture you can wear, as well as the size of your accessories.

PETITE

5ft 3in (1.60m) and under

- You're better wearing one color from head to toe
- Two colors may be worn as long as the proportions are $^2/_3$ to $^1/_3$
- Don't wear too much volume, as it will swamp you

Scale

You have:

- fine fingers, narrow wrists and ankles
- small facial features
- shoe size under 6 (37 EU)

You should wear:

- smaller print patterns
- smaller accessories
- minimal texture and bulk
- neat hairstyles

AVERAGE

5ft 3in–5ft 7in (1.60–1.70m)

- You have the freedom to do what you like, as long as you follow your body shape (pages 122–135) and proportions (pages 136–137)

Scale

You have:

- neither petite nor grand bone structure
- shoe size between 6 and 8 (37 and 40 EU)

You should wear:

- accessories that will balance your scale (neither tiny nor extra-large)
- average-sized patterns
- either a "wow" piece of clothing to make a statement or a single accessory such as a bag or a piece of jewelry

GRAND

5ft 7in (1.70m) and over

- You need to use color to break up your height
- By wearing differently proportioned clothes you will look more balanced (short jacket + short skirt will not do)

Scale

You have:

- large hands and feet, and strong bone structure
- shoe size 8+ (40+ EU)

You should wear:

- larger, bolder prints
- statement accessories
- heavier-weighted fabrics (or finer fabrics worn layered)

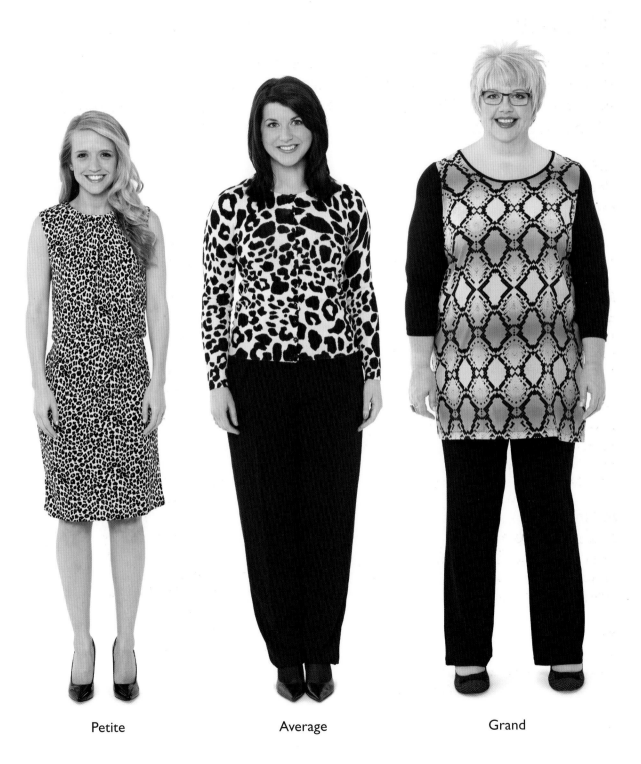

Petite   Average   Grand

FLATTERING COLOR

Now you know your best colors, you can combine them to create the look of a balanced body. Lighter or brighter colors will always draw attention to the areas where they're worn. Below are some of the most frequently used combinations.

ALL OVER COLOR

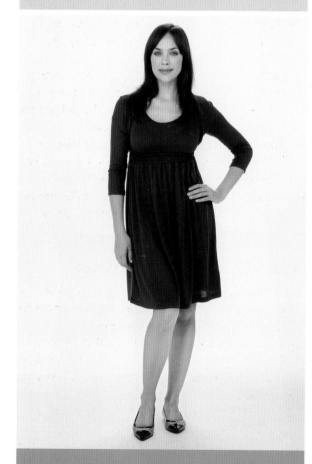

One color used for the entire outfit or a single-colored dress will give the appearance of height.

TWO COLORS

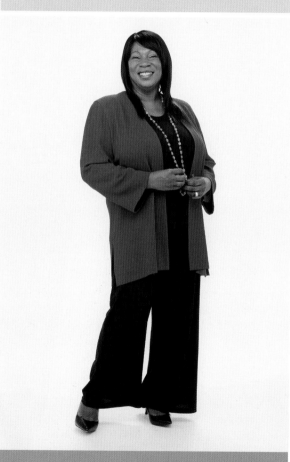

A jacket and skirt or pants in one color, with a top of another color, is a great combination for everybody.

COLOR BLOCKS

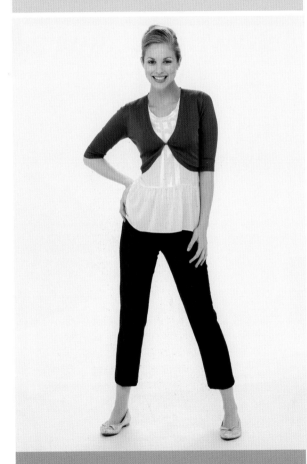

Different blocks of color on a jacket, top, skirt, or pants will give the appearance of reducing height.

CLEVER COMBINATIONS

You can use color to create an illusion of the perfect body shape, by using it creatively to alter "figure faults."

- **Full bust** Wear one of your darkest colors over your bust and add a lighter color, which may be worn over it.
- **Small bust** Wear a bright or light color here, adding embellishment over the bust if you like that kind of detail. Pockets are a good alternative. This will give the illusion of making your bust appear fuller.
- **Full hips or bottom** Use a dark color for skirts or pants; your dark neutrals or even black will work for most coloring types as it is away from the face.
- **Full waist** A striped or patterned top that finishes on the hips will take the eye away from the waist and draw attention to the hips.

OTHER WINNING COMBINATIONS

- A light top with a dark bottom will give the illusion of wider shoulders and slimmer hips, which is perfect for Triangles, but not for Inverted Triangles.
- A jacket in one color, with a top and skirt or pants in another, is a great combination for every body shape. If you are long in the body, you can break this look up with a belt.
- A dark top and light bottom will give the illusion of narrower shoulders and wider hips. This combination is excellent for Inverted Triangles, but not for Triangles; you need a light top and a darker bottom.

WHO CAN WEAR WHAT

By appreciating the subtle differences in the styling of clothes, you will be able to choose exactly the right type of jacket, skirt, top, and so on to flatter your body shape and so enhance your overall look. Be aware that some of the clothing details will need to change depending on your style personality.

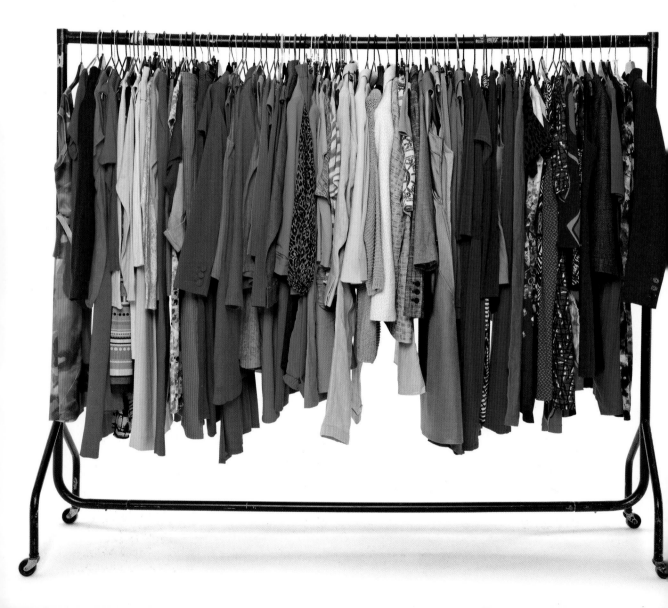

PANTS

Jeans

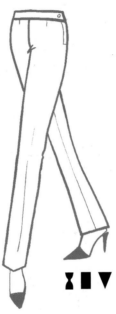

Narrow

Straight

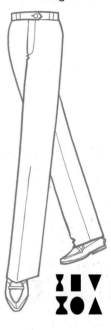

Plain front

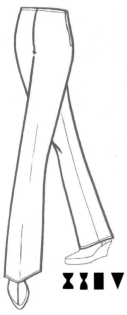

Drawstring

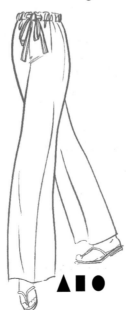

Cropped

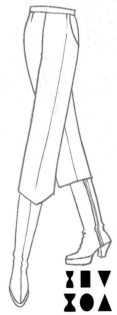

Note: Not with short full legs

SKIRTS

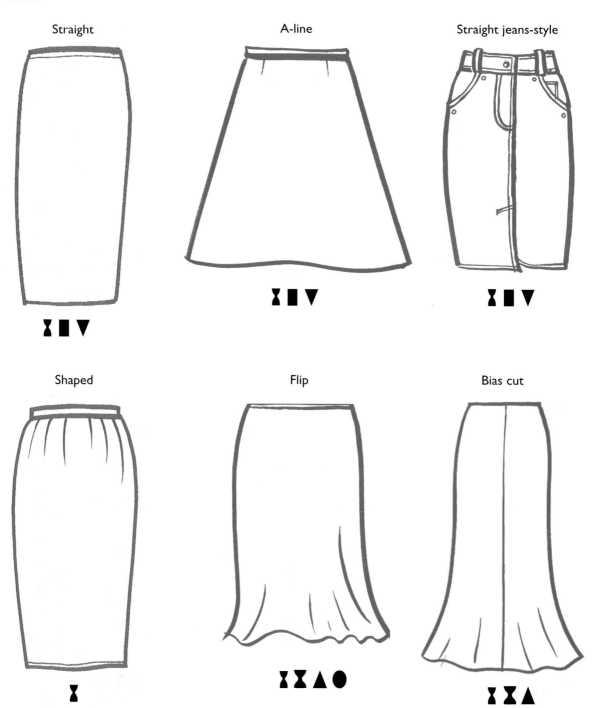

Straight

A-line

Straight jeans-style

Shaped

Flip

Bias cut

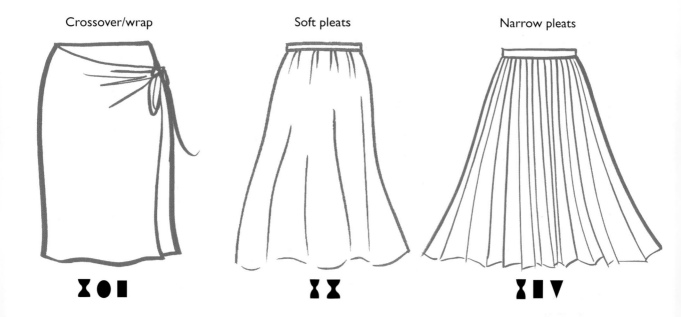

Crossover/wrap

Soft pleats

Narrow pleats

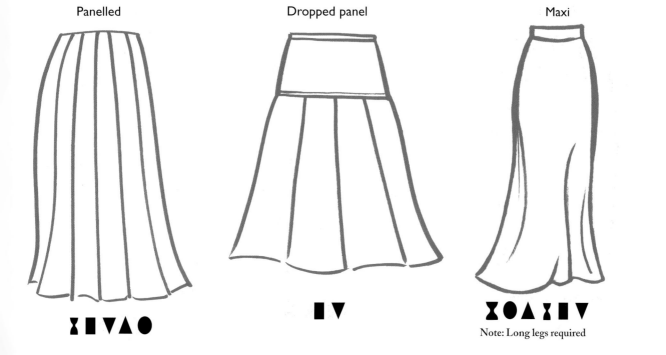

Panelled

Dropped panel

Maxi

Note: Long legs required

TOPS

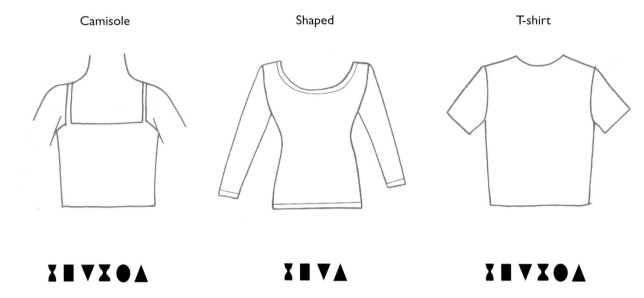

Camisole

Shaped

T-shirt

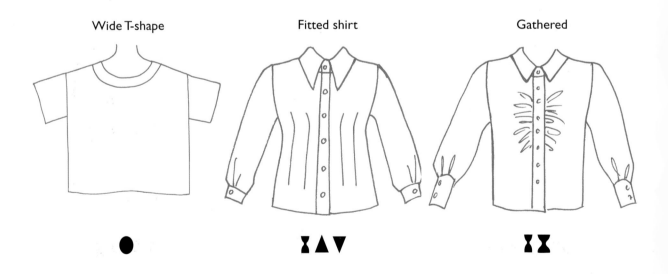

Wide T-shape

Fitted shirt

Gathered

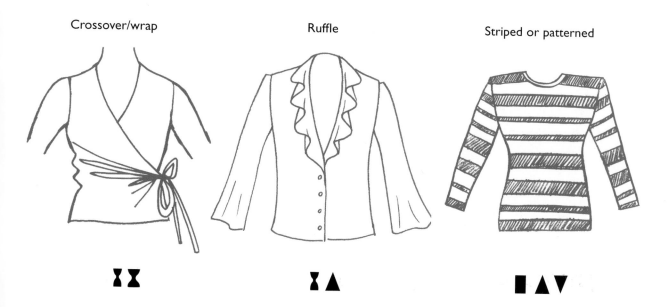

Crossover/wrap

Ruffle

Striped or patterned

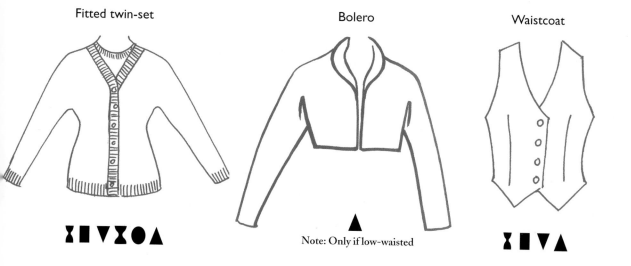

Fitted twin-set

Bolero

Note: Only if low-waisted

Waistcoat

JACKETS

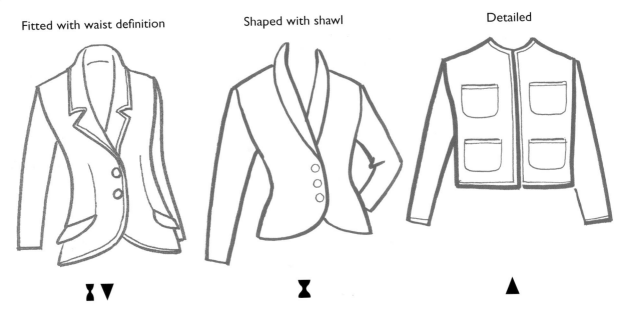

Fitted with waist definition

Shaped with shawl

Detailed

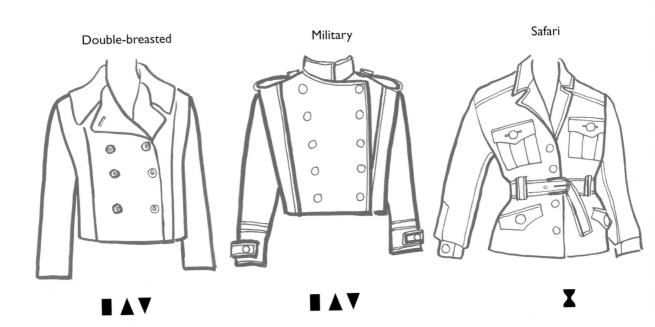

Double-breasted

Military

Safari

Biker

Fitted with peplum

Cropped

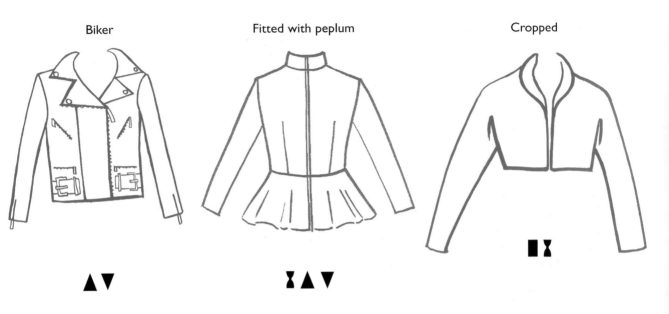

Waterfall

Deconstructed

Cardigan style

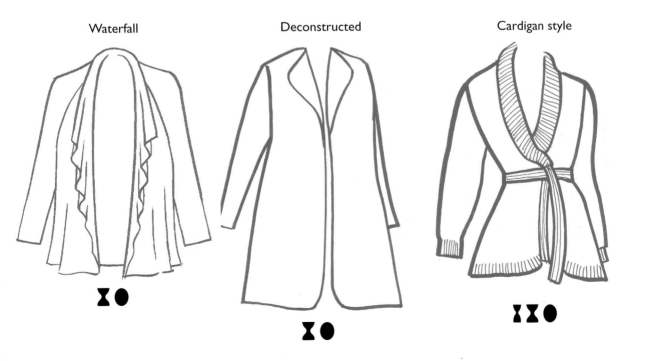

DRESSES

Straight shift

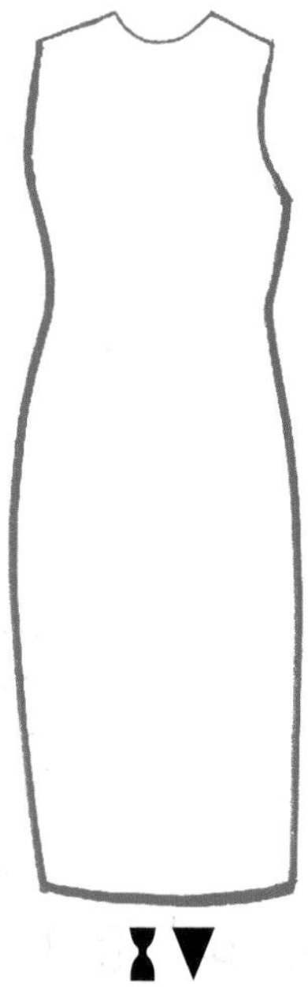

Fitted, belted shift

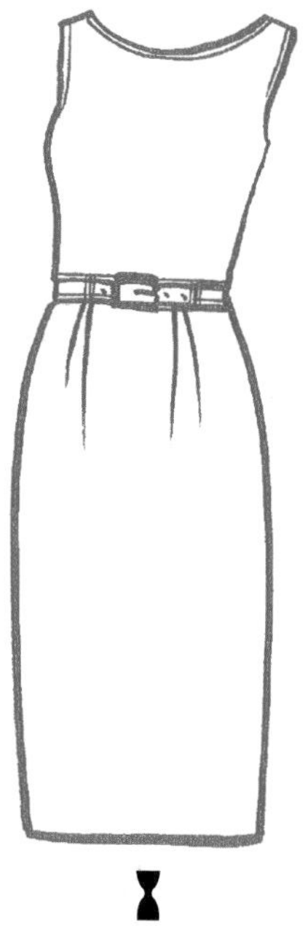

Shirt dress

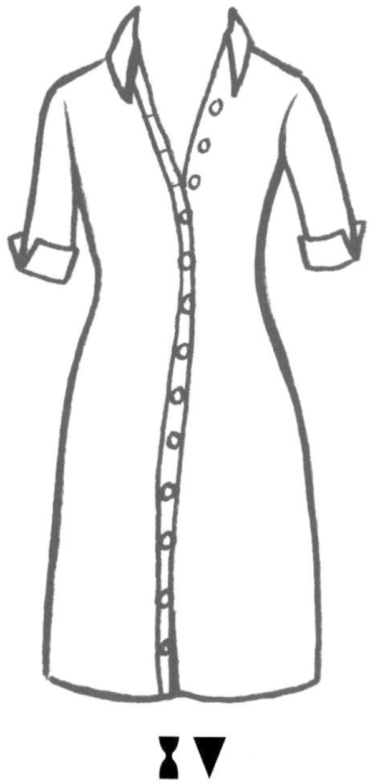

A-line

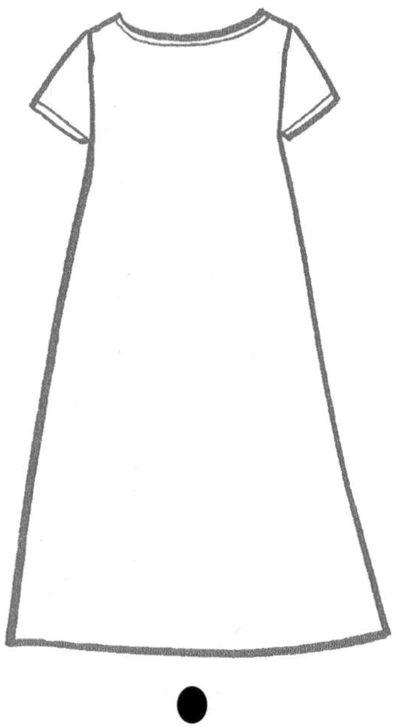

Princess line

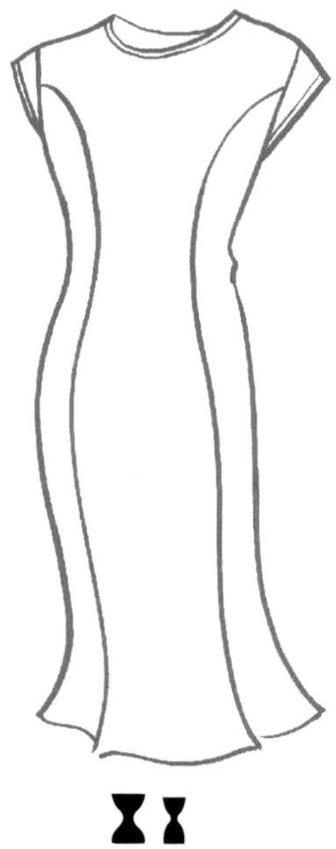

Bias cut

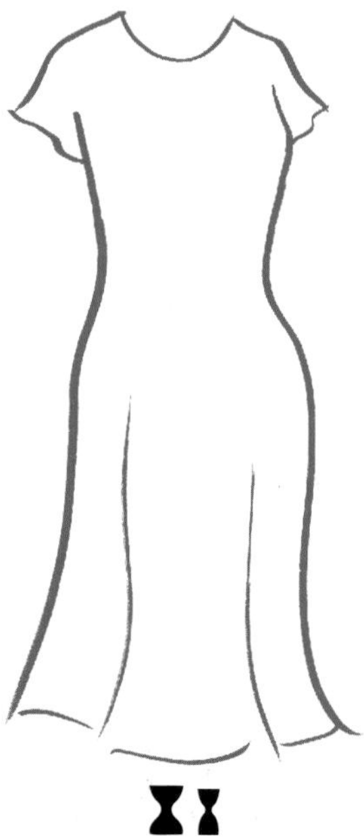

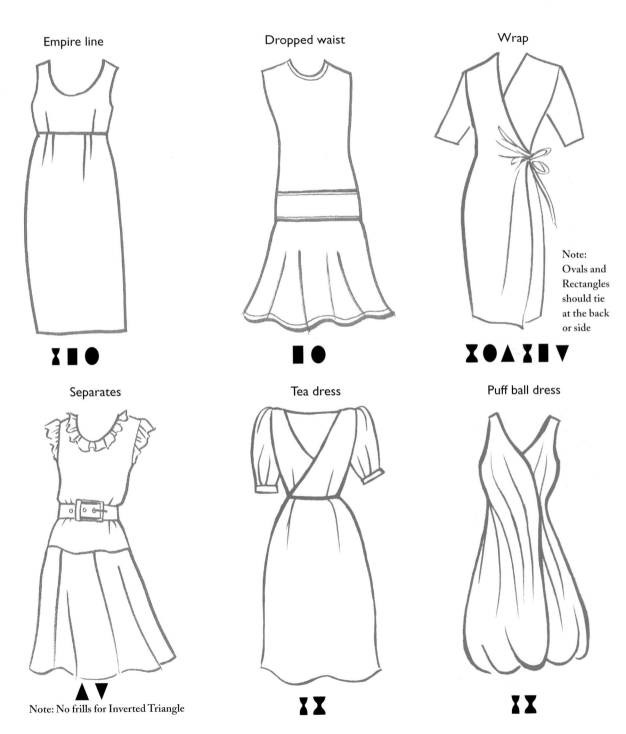

Empire line

Dropped waist

Wrap

Note:
Ovals and
Rectangles
should tie
at the back
or side

Separates

Tea dress

Puff ball dress

Note: No frills for Inverted Triangle

CLOTHING DETAILS

Your body shape and proportions will determine which clothing details, such as necklines, waistlines, and sleeves, will flatter you the most. By learning to look at your body objectively, you will know how to buy clothes to suit your shape.

THE GOLDEN RULE

There is one golden rule that will ensure you are showing off your body shape to your best advantage at all times: never finish any part of a garment at the widest point of your body. For example, you should avoid:

- jackets that finish at the widest point on your hips
- skirts that end at the fullest part of your legs
- short sleeves if you have a full bust
- short tops if you have a wide waist

NECKLINES

When deciding which necklines to wear, be aware of how prominent your collarbones and/or your upper chest are, and of how confident you feel to reveal these parts of your body.

- **Boat/slash** Gives the illusion of wide shoulders. Good for Triangle shapes, but avoid if you have prominent collarbones or a scrawny neck.
- **Bardot** Good for most shapes, but not if you have sloping shoulders.
- **V-necks** Look good on everyone, and can always be accessorized. Plunging V-necks are elegant—but not if you have a long neck or if they reveal too much cleavage.
- **Scoops** Work well on most women, particularly if you have narrow shoulders.
- **Cowl** Perfect for full busts and softer body lines.
- **Roll** Only if you have a long neck and no double chin or short neck.
- **Crew** Suits most women, but they need to sit well.
- **Ruffles/frills** Best for a longer neck and softer facial features.

- **Mandarin collars** Not for those with a short neck or double chin.
- **Shirt collars** Good for most women (unless short necked), and best worn open.
- **Jewel necklines** Good for all.
- **Halternecks** Excellent for Inverted Triangles.

BUST LINES

If you don't wear the right bra, your clothes won't hang properly: go to page 182—the wrong bra can alter your body shape and clothing size. Have a variety of bras to suit different occasions and different tops.

- **Small bust** Add details such as pockets, buttons, appliqué, ruffles, or slogans. Texture and layering are also helpful. A padded bra always helps.
- **Full bust** Stick to simple cuts and plain fabrics (no heavy textures). A V-neck or jewel neckline is best for you. Front-opening shirts and blouses need to be worn with care, and should be made of soft or stretchy fabric. A little ruching that will shape into the bust, or a crossover or wrap, will also work well. Make sure any darts in a garment fit underneath the fullest part of your bust.

SHOULDER LINES

- **Inserted** Good for all. If your shoulders slope or are rounded, consider shoulder pads.
- **Raglan** You need a square shoulder line to wear these successfully.
- **Dropped** Good for adding width to the shoulders. They will also soften a strong, straight shoulder line.
- **Shoulder pads** Great for straightening out sloping shoulders.

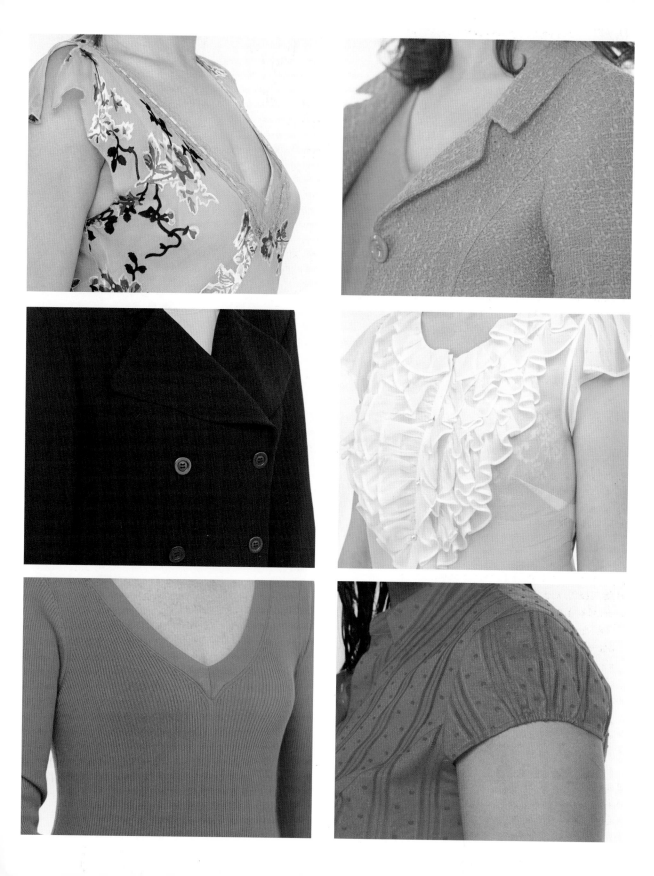

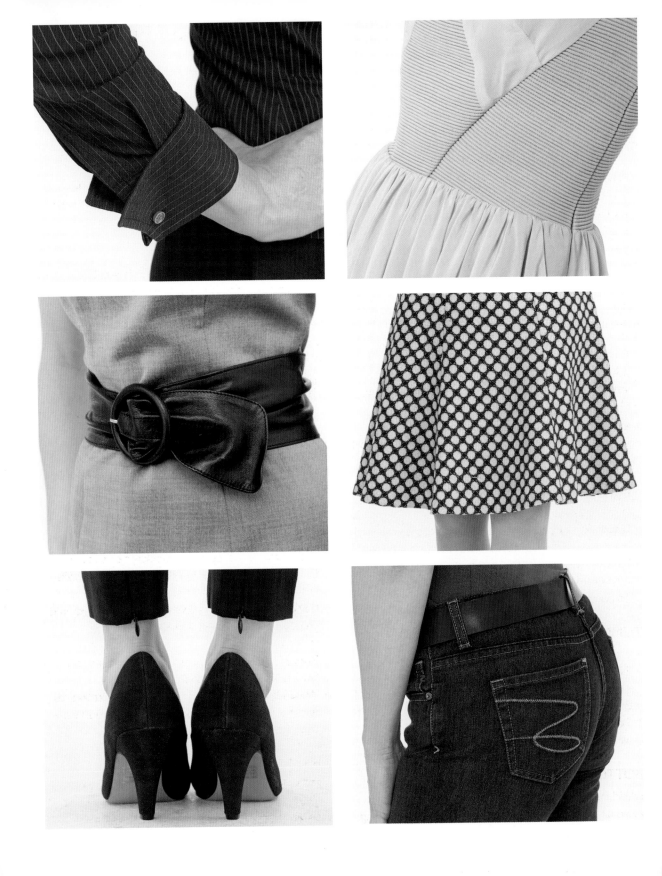

SLEEVES

The key factor when choosing a sleeve length is to remember never to end the sleeves at a wide point on your arm.
- **Bracelet** Great for short to average arms.
- **Full** Best for average to long arms.
- **Batwing** Best worn by average to tall women.
- **Cuff details** Make sure that these do not overwhelm your hands.

WAISTLINES

Create the illusion of a longer body by wearing a low waistline; to shorten your body, bring the waistline up.
- **Belts** Great for averting the eye from a full, rounded tummy.
- **Waistband** You need to have a clearly defined waist, as in Neat Hourglass, Full Hourglass, and Triangle shapes, to wear pants and skirts with waistbands. A wide waistband is excellent if you are long-waisted.
- **Elasticized** These may be your favorites if you have a fluctuating waistline. Best worn covered over, but beware of adding bulk. Non-gathered, elasticized waistbands are more flattering.
- **Dropped waist** Perfect for short-waisted women, but they don't work well for long-waisted women.
- **Hipsters** Good for short waists and those of you who do not have clearly defined waistlines (Inverted Triangles or Rectangles).

TUMMY LINES

- **Front pleats** Good if you have a flat tummy.
- **Zippers** Front zippers will add volume to your tummy; side and back zippers will give a sleeker look.
- **Pockets** Pockets with flaps suit women with flat hips. Sloping pockets and pockets without flaps can be worn by everyone.

BOTTOM LINES

Decide where the widest part of your bottom is and avoid any details in that area. Instead of wearing a long jacket or top to hide your bottom, show off an asset such as your waist.

THIGH LINES

If your thighs are wider than your hips, take care to avoid details in the thigh area. Looser-fitting pants and skirts are the answer.

HEMLINES

Most skirts and dresses are made to fit what manufacturers think is the average height (5ft 4in/ 1.65m). If you do not comply or do not have the most shapely legs it is important that you adjust the length to a flattering area of your leg. These rules also apply to pants, cut-offs, and shorts.
- **Above the knee** Most places will suit as long as the length is appropriate.
- **At the knee** At a narrow point on the knee, for most women this is just below the knee.
- **Calf length** Below fullest part.
- **Full length** At a narrow point of the ankle.

LEG LINES

- **Short legs** Wear skirts and pants with minimal volume. Open-fronted shoes with a short skirt will add length to the leg, as will stockings or socks in the same color as your pants or skirt. Avoid details and patterns.
- **Long legs** Wear skirts and pants with lots of volume and detail. Patterns and layers are good for you.
- **Skinny legs** Add volume with textured tights and fabrics. Avoid anything too clingy.
- **Wide legs** Wear the same color from waist to toes. Avoid anything too clingy or heavily textured. Loose and fluid fits work well.

ANKLE LINES

- **Thin** Add details such as ankle straps, socks, or different textures.
- **Wide** Go for open-fronted shoes.

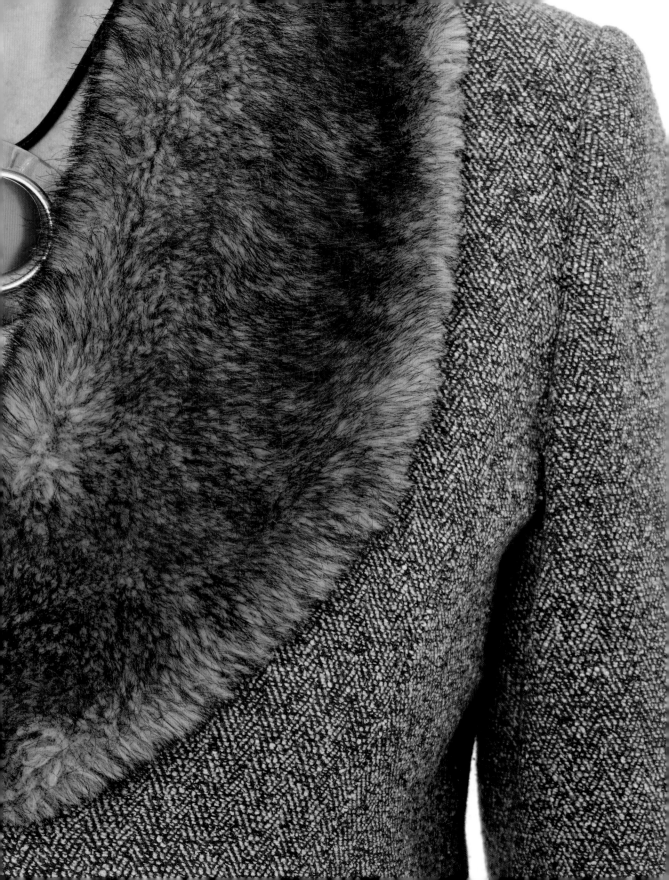

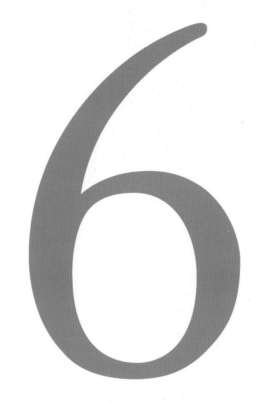

YOUR WORKING WARDROBE

WHAT DOES YOUR IMAGE SAY ABOUT YOU ?

The world of business has become more and more visual, whether it be the packaging, the marketing, or indeed what people choose to wear to conduct their business. It has been demonstrated that you have a mere 30 seconds in which to make a lasting impression.

Nearly 50 years ago, Professor Albert Mehrabian (*Silent Messages*, 1971 and 1985) reported that 55 percent of how somebody judges us come from signals we give out and our appearance; 38 percent is how we sound: the tone, the pitch, and the pace of our voice; and only 7 percent is about the actual words we say.

For the past 25 years we have worked with all types of companies helping men and women at all levels with their careers to develop their personal image in a way that is appropriate for their career, age, and

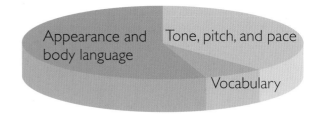

the industry they are working in. We know that if someone feels confident about their look, their body language will become more positive and open and they will sound in control.

Your image will undoubtedly affect your performance. If you look good and feel good and in control you will attract recognition from others.

BODY LANGUAGE

Body language is the silent messages we send out to others. The way we stand, our posture, how we use our hands, our eye contact, our facial expressions, our special awareness of others, and our grooming are all the signals that others pick up instinctively. If you feel that you are not always coming across in the most positive manner, maybe you need to have some advice on your body language and behavior pattern. Alternatively, you may choose to refer to Allan Pease's *The Definitive Book of Body Language*.

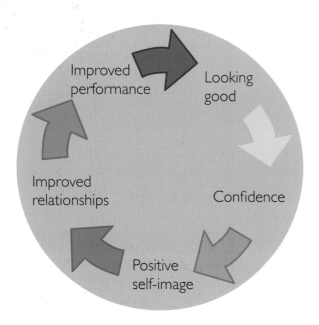

YOUR VOICE

When you feel under-confident, the tone, the pitch, and the pace of the voice reflects how you feel. Women's voices can become raised and squeaky, the words can become jumbled (because they are panicking and speaking too quickly), and the tone will become monotone (no intonation). One easy way of improving the tone of your voice is to speak aloud to others (recording your own voice to hear how you sound, or even reading a story to children). To improve the pace, think about the punctuation in a sentence and pause when there should be a comma or a period. The pitch is improved by being enthusiastic and believing in what you are talking about.

YOUR APPEARANCE

Wearing clothes that complement you, and are appropriate for your job, will give you confidence and you will notice that your stance and your posture will improve too.

In Chapter 1 (see pages 12–19) of this book we recommend that you analyze your clothes and lifestyle to establish the priorities in your wardrobe. A wardrobe that works for you is one that reflects your lifestyle and the type of work you do. When setting a budget for your clothes, you should spend the most on the items that you wear the most. Good investment pieces can be styled and updated with the latest accessories.

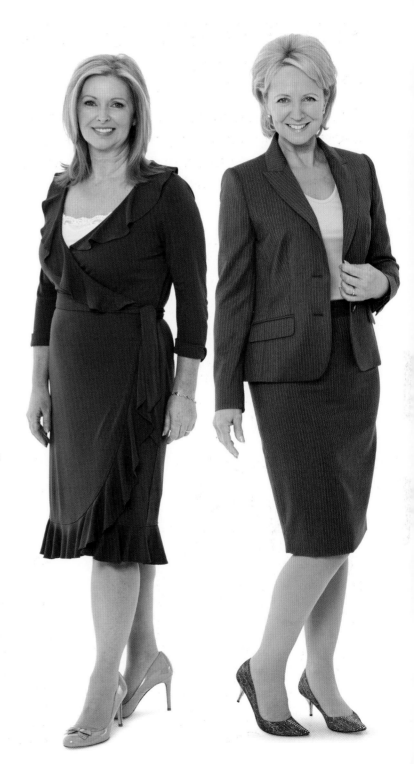

THE CAREER LADDER

Dress for the job you want, not for the job you are in. If you look the part, people will believe that you can do the job. It's all about nonverbal signals, creating the brand "YOU," and standing out from the crowd.

DEVELOPING YOUR BRAND

Your image is made up of your personality, attitude, behavior, habits, education, and personal values. This does not mean, of course, that qualifications and experience are not relevant, but to stand out in a competitive market you need to differentiate yourself from your colleagues using your communication skills and personal image.

DRESSING FOR AN INTERVIEW

You will be short-listed for an interview on the strength of your qualifications and experience. Once that has happened, you need to impress the interviewer. You need to identify the brand values of the organization you hope to work for. Research the company to find out if it is traditional in its attitude, at the cutting edge of technology, or friendly? You need to ensure that you reflect those values. The list below gives some guidelines as to what you should consider when planning what to wear for an interview.

- **Law firm** Formal, professional, traditional
- **Cutting edge** Business casual and current
- **Friendly** Business casual, think approachable colors
- **Health care** Impeccable grooming

Dress codes will differ from company to company, so it's a good idea, if you have the opportunity, to stand outside the organization during a lunch hour to observe what the existing staff are wearing.

Always err on the side of caution—it is better to be more formally dressed than too casual.

CLIMBING THE CAREER LADDER

Once you have a job, you'll want to make your mark and be noticed for promotion to the next level. This means that you can't revert to your pre-interview wardrobe; instead you need to build on the brand that got you the job in the first place. You will need to conform to the dress code of the organization and ensure that your grooming is impeccable. This will give the impression that you are organized and totally efficient. Someone who cannot wash her hair in the morning or put her makeup on will not portray efficiency and organizational skills. It is a good idea to aspire to dress like someone you value for their business appearance and skills within your workplace.

RETURNING TO WORK

A large number of women return to work after a career break due to pregnancy or looking after an elderly relative. During their time away from work, it is possible that they may have gained some weight, not bought many clothes, or have lost confidence compared to their peers who have kept on working.

Returning to work is the time to assess your style personality, colors, and your body shape to make sure that your re-entry into the workplace is as smooth and stress free as possible. Your new image needs to reflect the fact that you may have a young family to organize before stepping out of the door. Consider a low-maintenance hairstyle, a well-coordinated wardrobe, and a simple but effective makeup routine that you can do in no more than 15 minutes.

WORKING LATER IN LIFE

It used to be that once a woman reached her fifties, retirement was around the corner. Not anymore! Women live longer, the retirement age is increasing, and many women are no longer willing to give up an enjoyable and/or remunerative job just because of their age. The major challenge these women face is understanding how to keep their look updated without dressing too "young."

You will probably have a closet full of clothes but perhaps you need to retire some items and replace them with more current pieces. Women's fashion trends run in a five-year cycle, so examine anything that you have had in your closet for more than six years and ask yourself whether it is still current.

GUIDELINES

- **Hairstyle** Color and cut appropriate and reviewed regularly
- **Skirt length** Not too long, not too short
- **Pants** Appropriate style
- **Jackets** It is not enough to keep it just because it still fits
- **Accessories** Current—there is nothing more dating than "old fashioned" accessories

Try to keep pace with technology. You do not have to become an expert but an awareness will ensure you are not at a disadvantage with your younger colleagues.

COLORS IN THE WORKPLACE

Refer to your dominant palette. Whatever the darker colors in your palette are, they will portray authority. High contrast is also authoritative. Medium-depth colors and a tonal look will always be more approachable and less threatening. Light colors will have no credibility in a formal environment but are fun and interesting in a more casual workplace. See pages 44–47 for more about color psychology.

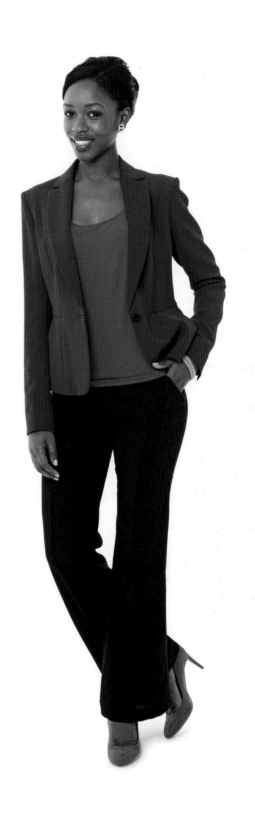

KEEPING YOUR WARDROBE CURRENT

Whether you are a returner, looking for a new career, or a promotion with your current employers, it is important that your look is not only suitable for your coloring, body shape, and industry, but also current—an out-of-date look will give the impression that your work ethic and ideas are also dated.

This does not mean constantly changing your wardrobe and being a fashion victim, but keeping abreast of trends. In Creating a Capsule Wardrobe (see pages 170–177) we suggest that you invest in basic pieces in neutral colors—these will probably need to be updated on a regular basis. As already mentioned, trends in women's fashions tend to go in five-year cycles, so you will need to assess any garment that you've had for longer than this, to ensure that it is still current and conveys a sense of stylish modernity.

Make it a habit to audit your wardrobe regularly. The best time to do so is probably at the change of season. Be strict with yourself and do a constructive closet clear-out (see Organizing Your Closet, pages 188–189).

Hairstyle

When was the last time you changed your hairstyle? If you have had the same style for more than five years, it may be time for a change. What about freshening up the color? A semipermanent tint, highlights, or lowlights will always give an updated look to any style; but stay within your color palette range or be aware that if you dramatically change your hair color, you may need to change your coloring type too. Be prepared that if you color your hair, it will require maintenance and regular visits to the hairdresser.

Jackets

Jacket lengths alter and the wrong length jacket will definitely date your look. Collar size and shape also change regularly, so make sure yours do not date the jacket—and you in the process.

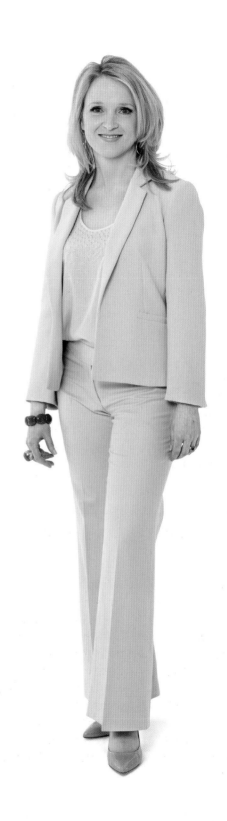

Skirts

Whatever the length, make sure skirts end at a slim point of your leg—usually just below the knee or just below the calf. There are always subtle changes to the shape of skirts, from straight to A-line, pleated, narrow, or box pleats, for example. Whatever the trend, make sure the shape works for you and if it doesn't, look for an alterative such as a dress or pants in the right style for you.

Pants

Consider pant width and rise length—low-rise pants are good if you are short in the rise, but if you are not they will not be suitable for the workplace.

Shoes

Think about what shoe shapes are available, and what is best for you: pointed (will elongate your legs), rounded, or with square toes. How much walking do you need to do? What about changing to more suitable shoes when you get to your place of work? Remember, you'll need different styles in your closet to match your outfits. For example, with an elegant wrap dress you will not want to wear loafers.

Boots

Again, you'll want different styles for different looks and different occasions. To lengthen the leg, wear stockings/pantyhose the same color as your boots.

Handbags

Your handbag is as important as any other item of your look. Make sure it balances with your scale and is suitable for its task. If you have to carry items to a meeting, can your handbag fulfill this purpose or do you need something else to carry your laptop and papers in? A shopping bag is never appropriate for this job. Handbags can be fun and often they are great to use as a pop of color in your overall look. Opt for a classic style to ensure longevity, but make sure it is modern enough to demonstrate you know what's what!

PERSONAL PRESENTATION

- Your hands play a major part in communication so it is essential they are well groomed. Long red talons may be fun but a French manicure or softer colors may be more suitable in a male-dominated industry. As always make sure the color is appropriate. There are many different manicures available and techniques such as gel nails/everlasting manicures give a long-lasting look that is great for busy working women.
- Make sure your personal freshness, achieved by regular bathing or showering, is impeccable. Be sure you are always pleasant to be near by changing your deodorant on a regular basis because you can build up immunity if you use just one brand constantly.
- Use breath fresheners if you smoke or tend to eat spicy foods.
- Change your clothes and shoes daily to keep them looking fresh—nothing is worse than perspiring afresh onto stale clothes.
- Place clothes on good-quality hangers at the end of the day. This will prevent your garments becoming wrinkled.
- Visit the dental hygienist regularly.
- Choose you perfume with care—a light daytime fragrance is the most suitable. The general guideline is the fragrance is on you and should not remain in the room after you have left. Avoid heavy musky or heavy floral perfumes. Light citrus or natural floral eau de toilette are the safest bet.

WHAT TO AVOID

- Showing too much flesh
- Flashy jewelry or large statement designer logo pieces
- Shoes you can't walk well in
- Faded or worn-out items of clothing
- Sportswear of any kind in the workplace, unless appropriate
- Visible body or facial piercings
- Visible body tattoos

CASE STUDY: FORMAL

Meet Ann; she's a Dramatic (see pages 28–29). Her style can leap from Romantic to Creative as the mood takes her. She is an avid shopper, collecting accessories and unusual pieces around the world. However, her academic performances have led her to a serious professional career.

PROFESSIONAL BRANDING

Ann was asked to list the core brand values of her business and how she wished to be seen by her clients and competitors. We then suggested how these values should be reflected in her wardrobe.

- **Dynamic** Ann needs to make a statement but it needs to be appropriate for the industries she is working in.
- **In control** To give the appearance of being in control; Ann needs to be neat and tidy.
- **Works with men** Ann is petite in height and stature, so needs to demonstrate that she is in control, particularly when working with men. She therefore needs a fairly formal approach to her clothing choices; the colors she wears have to be in neutral shades and the kind that men feel comfortable with in the workplace.
- **Professional** Ann's clothing style needs to be appropriate for the industry she is working in and therefore a formal look, in neutral shades again, will work best. She will not display flesh, she will wear pantyhose in the summer and her shoes and other accessories will be current but understated.
- **Knowledgeable** Confident body language and good eye contact will ensure that Ann displays her knowledge and she knows her subject inside out to those she is working with.
- **Approachable** Using medium-depth colors mixed with neutrals will not only give Ann authority but also show that she is approachable.

THE MAKEOVER

Ann's first look is how she loves to dress. She wears a feminine dress with a belt that is really a bow, flowers on her cardigan, and a very dramatic color combination between the cream dress and the red cardigan, stockings, and shoes. Her shoes are high fashion and the red stockings and shoes will actually draw attention away from her face, her eyes, and her lovely smile. Facial expressions and eye contact are vital in business—they are how people judge your performance and how confident and knowledgeable you are. The color blocking in this look actually makes Ann appear shorter, which has the effect of diminishing her overall impact. The choice of red can also be seen as aggressive and unapproachable (see page 44).

In her second look, Ann is wearing appropriate colors for a formal work look. The taupe dress is approachable yet business like. Her stylish jacket is striking but once again in appropriate colors. The details of the jacket will appeal to Ann's fashion flair but will not distract from the message she is presenting.

The shoes tone with the outfit and because the dress is light all the attention will be on Ann's face (not her legs and shoes). We always say "build your image to the face, that's how we communicate with others."

Careful, appropriate dressing is a vital part of your business image along with all the other aspects of how others judge us.

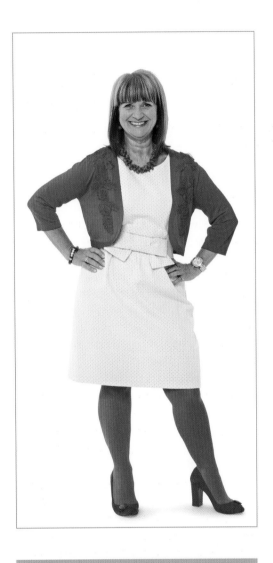

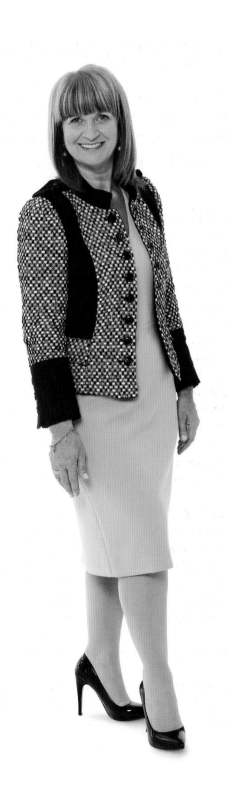

ANN'S STATISTICS
- Coloring: Warm
- Scale: Petite
- Body shape: Triangle
- Proportions: Long rise + short legs

CASE STUDY: BUSINESS CASUAL

Anna's career for the past two decades has been as a senior executive within a global fast-moving consumer goods company. She traveled widely and was often presenting new products and concepts to large audiences. Her image was formal, authoritative, and controlling. After a lifestyle change (and wedding bells) she has re-trained as a life coach and her image needs to be approachable, friendly, and nonthreatening, but still very much in control.

PROFESSIONAL BRANDING

Anna is in her early fifties but will be dealing with men and women of all ages, so needs to look current, innovative, and forward thinking in her approach and image. Again, we asked Anna what message she wanted to give out now that she has switched careers. Here are the results together with some guidelines on her new workwear.

- **Approachable** By wearing colors in medium shades, Anna will look approachable and nonthreatening. The darker the shades she wears, the more forbidding she will appear.
- **Friendly** Interesting, fashionable, and less formal clothes will always be more friendly than a formal business suit, which creates a barrier between Anna and her clients.
- **Knowledgeable** Confident body language and great energy levels will give the impression of knowledge. Mature women need to keep current with their look; maturity will more often than not portray confidence and knowledge, however if the image is dated clients will assume that the knowledge is dated too!
- **Trustworthy** This is demonstrated by good eye contact; if you can't look someone in the eye it will be assumed that you have something to hide.
- **Nonthreatening** Open friendly gestures, giving people their own space, and having a relaxed stance will all give the impression of being nonthreatening. Don't forget to smile—a real smile, not a forced one.

THE MAKEOVER

In her first look, Anna is wearing the typical black business pantsuit. She wears it with the ubiquitous white blouse making the whole outfit a severe, unapproachable, and threatening one. Black is the most authoritative color anyone can wear and when teamed with white, the contrast is even more forbidding. The black handbag looks like a briefcase and Anna resembles a lawyer going off to court, not someone who is there to listen, be empathetic, and give guidance. She looks like she is about to distribute rules and strict guidelines! As Anna is Soft she'll need to wear harsher makeup colors to balance her soft tone with the strength of the black-and-white outfit.

In her second look, Anna has completely changed the style of her look. The colors complement her soft coloring and her makeup is now softer and more natural. The dress and cardigan combination is friendly, approachable, and yet fashionable. The colors are totally non-threatening and the soft pattern is informal but still business like. Everything about Anna's look is friendly and comfortable. She looks relaxed and her outfit is suitable for her to wear as she coaches someone, whether male or female, either in their home or in an office environment.

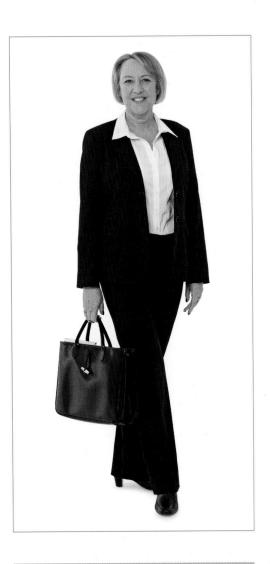

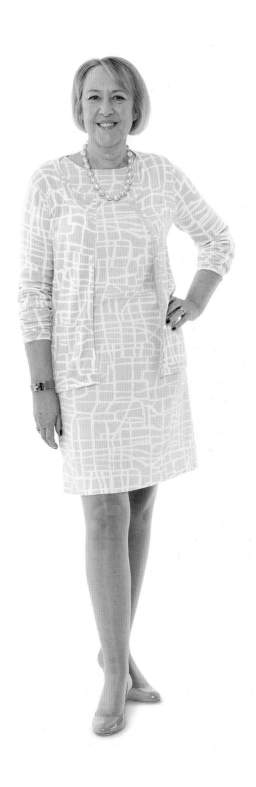

ANNA'S STATISTICS
- Coloring: Soft
- Scale: Average
- Body shape: Neat Hourglass
- Proportions: High waist + long legs

CASE STUDY: CASUAL

Marie's career in a male-orientated national industry meant her work wardrobe was functional rather than fashionable and relaxed; she was often called to be on site where health and safety were an issue. After a career break, Marie decided to change direction and now works for an alzheimer's charity, since a close family member is a sufferer.

PROFESSIONAL BRANDING

Marie's wardrobe now is simply casual and practical. She is now working within a charitable environment so her peers are often relaxed in their choice of clothes. Wearing a casual look for work means you can be comfortable, but not sloppy.

- **Friendly** Marie now needs to get away from the darkest shades of her palette, or wear these in contrast with some fun colors, to demonstrate how approachable and friendly she is. Any colors signaling aggression should not be in her wardrobe.
- **Empathetic** Marie will take her cue for her new dress code from her patients and their visitors, so non-showy or nonthreatening outfits are necessary.
- **Caring** Her body language will be sympathetic and open, whether she is dealing with the patients or with their families.
- **Fun** The advice we gave Marie is to go for the brighter shades of her palette. When you wear color, people tend to smile and respond positively. Wearing a stripy top always looks fun and friendly.
- **Budget-conscious** With a new lifestyle, comes a new budget, and a lower one at that. Marie will pick inexpensive pieces in comfortable fabrics that are easy to move in, and that can be taken off easily.
- **Low maintenance** Days of mani-pedi may be over, or at least of going to a salon to have them done. Now, since she still needs to be groomed and must make sure her appearance is neat and tidy, she will do these herself.

THE MAKEOVER

Marie's first look is how she used to dress for business in her previous career. She worked alongside male colleagues and her work wardrobe needed to be businesslike and functional, although she liked to retain her feminine side. She made site visits, so her clothes needed to be simple to ensure that nothing could cause a safety hazard.

In her new career, Marie is called upon to do all kinds of caring. She must be able to move easily; she may need to kneel, sit on the floor, run, jump, and even lift patients. She never knows what condition her patients may be in, so her clothes need to be low maintenance. We have dressed her in a relaxed T-shirt in cheerful deep and bright colors. Stripes are fun and stimulating as well. Marie has an amazing Inverted Triangle figure so stripes suit her well, and because of her narrow hips she will always look stunning in jeans (she can certainly take all the details on her hips). The flat sneakers she is wearing make it easy for her to stand on her feet all day if need be.

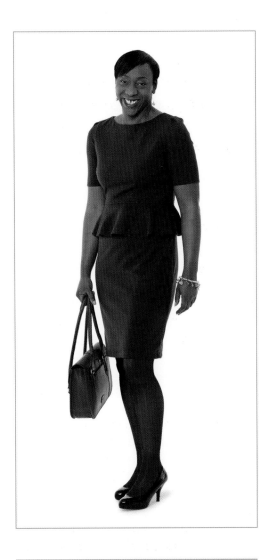

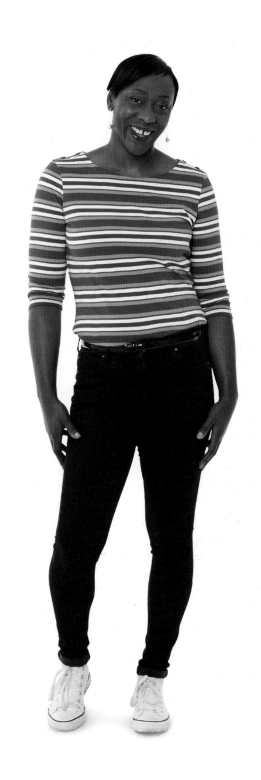

MARIE'S STATISTICS
- Coloring: Deep
- Scale: Grand
- Body shape: Inverted Triangle
- Proportions: Long rise + long legs

CREATING A CAPSULE WARDROBE

Before deciding how many items you want in your capsule wardrobe you need to assess your body shape and any figure challenges (for example, front-opening shirts are not suitable for fuller busts). Your formal wardrobe should consist of two to three neutral colors from your basic color palette, with fashion colors added for tops and accessories when appropriate.

On the opposite page we have suggested six colors for a capsule wardrobe, three neutrals and three fashion colors. Then, on the following pages we have taken each body shape and, using just 12 pieces, we have assembled 24 outfits that will take you from a formal business wardrobe to a business casual and even a casual look. We have labeled the garments that should be purchased in neutral colors to give you a flexible and workable capsule wardrobe. The colors may be varied according to lifestyle, time of year, and suitability for the workplace. Remember investments buys are always best in neutral colors.

This is just a guide to help you put a capsule wardrobe together. It is a good idea to do a closet clear out before you start as you will probably find that you have some of the garments in appropriate colors already. You then just need to add the complementary ones to start to build your capsule wardrobe. Don't forget to personalize your image with your own accessories to develop your look in harmony with your style personality.

Anyone at any level can still wear casual clothes and be businesslike. It will depend on what you do and where you work. A business casual wardrobe is exactly what it says. It is businesslike but more informal and relaxed than a formal wardrobe. Business suits may be replaced with a cardigan or colored jacket. Business casual presents a good opportunity to mix and match; maybe try some of the formal clothes you have in

your closet with some of the pieces you usually wear outside work. This is an easier wardrobe to work in harmony and balance with your style personality and body shape.

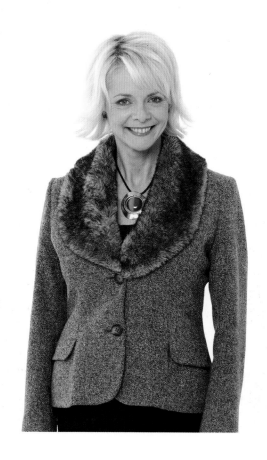

LIGHT CAPSULE

NEUTRAL	FASHION
Cocoa	Dusty Rose
Pewter	Light Aqua
Ivory	Sky Blue

DEEP CAPSULE

NEUTRAL	FASHION
Black	Soft White
Charcoal	True Red
Purple	Teal

WARM CAPSULE

NEUTRAL	FASHION
Olive	Lime
Cream	Terracotta
Chocolate	Primrose

COOL CAPSULE

NEUTRAL	FASHION
Charcoal	Light Teal
Dark Navy	Bright Periwinkle
Cassis	Icy Blue

CLEAR CAPSULE

NEUTRAL	FASHION
Black	Ivory
Royal Blue	Emerald Turquoise
Scarlet	Duck Egg

SOFT CAPSULE

NEUTRAL	FASHION
Taupe	Blush Pink
Stone	Jade
Rose Brown	Charcoal Blue

NEAT HOURGLASS CAPSULE

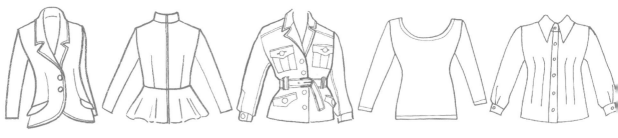

1 Fitted jacket with waist definition (neutral)

2 Fitted jacket with peplum (neutral)

3 Safari jacket (neutral)

4 Shaped top

5 Fitted shirt

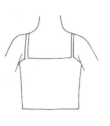

6 Camisole (neutral)

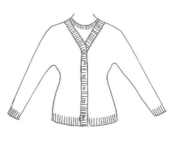

7 a & b Fitted twin-set

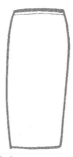

8 Straight skirt (neutral)

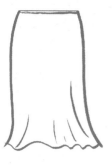

9 Flip skirt (neutral)

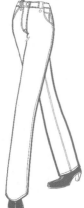

10 Classic jeans

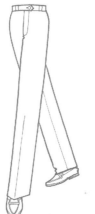

11 Straight pants (neutral)

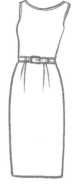

12 Fitted, belted shift dress

FORMAL CAPSULE

1 + 8 + 4
2 + 11 + 5
12 + 1
2 + 8 + 6
1 + 9 + 6
12 + 2
1 + 11 + 6
2 + 9 + 7b

BUSINESS CASUAL CAPSULE

9 + 7 a & b
11 + 4
12 + 7a
8 + 5
12
8 + 7
11 + 7
8 + 4

CASUAL CAPSULE

10 + 6 + 7a
10 + 5
11 + 6 + 3
9 + 4
12 + 3
10 + 4
11 + 3 + 4
10 + 6

For fabrics refer to pages 124–125.

FULL HOURGLASS CAPSULE

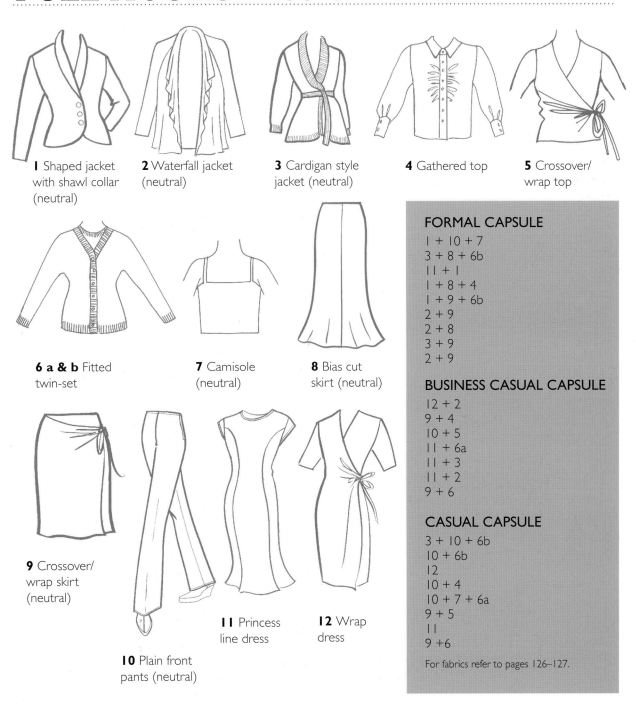

1 Shaped jacket with shawl collar (neutral)

2 Waterfall jacket (neutral)

3 Cardigan style jacket (neutral)

4 Gathered top

5 Crossover/ wrap top

6 a & b Fitted twin-set

7 Camisole (neutral)

8 Bias cut skirt (neutral)

9 Crossover/ wrap skirt (neutral)

10 Plain front pants (neutral)

11 Princess line dress

12 Wrap dress

FORMAL CAPSULE

1 + 10 + 7
3 + 8 + 6b
11 + 1
1 + 8 + 4
1 + 9 + 6b
2 + 9
2 + 8
3 + 9
2 + 9

BUSINESS CASUAL CAPSULE

12 + 2
9 + 4
10 + 5
11 + 6a
11 + 3
11 + 2
9 + 6

CASUAL CAPSULE

3 + 10 + 6b
10 + 6b
12
10 + 4
10 + 7 + 6a
9 + 5
11
9 + 6

For fabrics refer to pages 126–127.

TRIANGLE CAPSULE

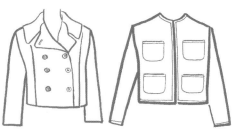

1 Double-breasted jacket (neutral)

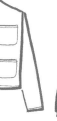

2 Detailed jacket (neutral)

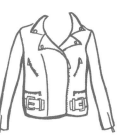

3 Biker jacket (neutral)

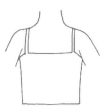

4 Camisole (neutral)

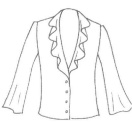

5 Ruffle top

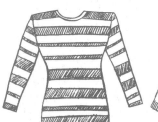

6 Striped or patterned top

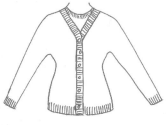

7 a & b Fitted Twin-set

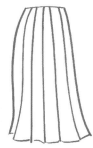

8 Paneled skirt (neutral)

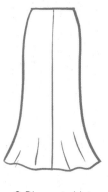

9 Bias-cut skirt (neutral)

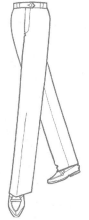

10 Straight pants

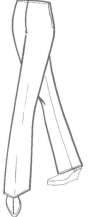

11 Plain front pants (neutral)

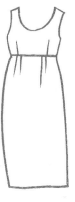

12 Empire line dress

FORMAL CAPSULE

1 + 10 + 4
2 + 8 + 7b
12 + 2
1 + 8 + 4
1 + 9 + 4
1 + 11 + 7b
3 + 11 + 7b

BUSINESS CASUAL CAPSULE

9 + 6
11 + 5
8 + 6
8 + 5
9 + 5
9 + 7b
11 + 7
11 + 6
12 + 7a
12

CASUAL CAPSULE

10 + 7b + 3
11 + 6
9 + 4 + 7a
9 + 5
10 + 5
10 + 4 + 3
9 + 4 + 3

For fabrics refer to pages 128–129.

OVAL CAPSULE

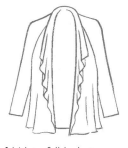

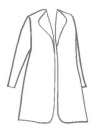

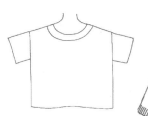

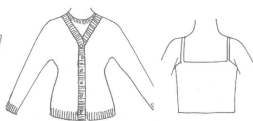

1 Waterfall jacket (neutral)

2 Deconstructed jacket (neutral)

3 Wide T-shape top (neutral)

4 a & b Twin-set

5 Camisole

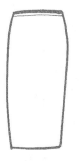

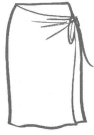

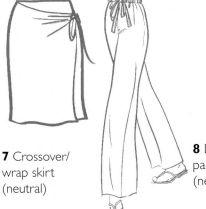

6 Straight skirt (neutral)

7 Crossover/ wrap skirt (neutral)

8 Drawstring pants (neutral)

FORMAL CAPSULE

1 + 6 + 3
2 + 9 + 5
11 + 2
1 + 7 + 5
1 + 9 + 4b
2 + 8 + 4b
2 + 9 + 4b

BUSINESS CASUAL CAPSULE

7 + 3
8 + 4
9 + 5
3 + 9
3 + 8
3 + 6
4 + 7
4 + 9
12
11

CASUAL CAPSULE

10 + 4a
12 + 9
6 + 3
8 + 5 + 4a
7 + 4
10
9+ 3

For fabrics refer to pages 130–131.

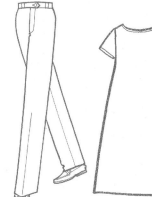

9 Straight pants (neutral)

10 A-line dress (neutral)

11 Empire line dress

12 Wrap dress

RECTANGLE CAPSULE

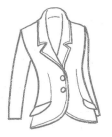

1 Fitted jacket with waist definition (neutral)

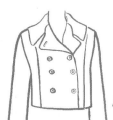

2 Double-breasted jacket (neutral)

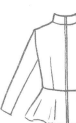

3 Fitted jacket with peplum (neutral)

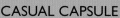

4 Shaped top

5 Fitted shirt

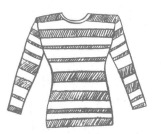

6 Striped or patterned top

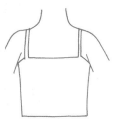

7 Camisole (neutral)

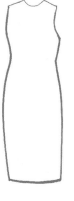

8 Straight skirt (neutral)

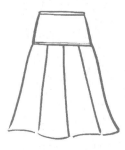

9 Dropped panel skirt (neutral)

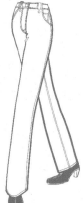

10 Jeans (neutral)

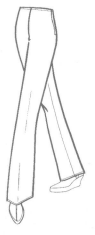

11 Plain front pants (neutral)

12 Straight shift dress (neutral)

FORMAL CAPSULE
1 + 8 + 4
2 + 9 + 6
12 + 3
3 + 8 + 7
1 + 9 + 6
1 + 11 + 6
2 + 10 + 7
2 + 9 + 4
2 + 9 + 7

BUSINESS CASUAL CAPSULE
9 + 6
11 + 5
8 + 4
12
11 + 6
8 + 5
9 + 5
9 + 4

CASUAL CAPSULE
10 + 7 + 6
11 + 4
9 + 6
10 + 7 + 3
10 + 4
10 + 5
10 + 7 + 2

For fabrics refer to pages 132–133.

INVERTED TRIANGLE CAPSULE

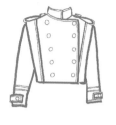

1 Military jacket (neutral)

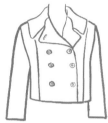

2 Double-breasted jacket (neutral)

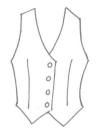

3 Vest (neutral)

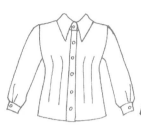

4 Fitted shirt

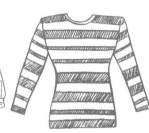

5 Striped or patterned top (neutral)

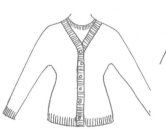

6 a & b Fitted twin-set

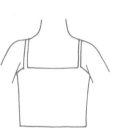

7 Camisole (neutral)

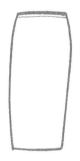

8 Straight skirt (neutral)

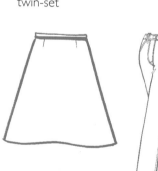

9 A-line skirt (neutral)

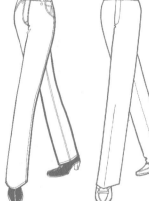

10 Classic jeans **11** Straight pants (neutral)

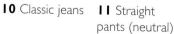

12 Fitted, belted shift dress

FORMAL CAPSULE

1 + 11 + 7
2 + 9 + 6b
11 + 3 + 4
12 + 2
1 + 8 + 7
1 + 8 + 5
2 + 11 + 5
2 + 8 + 6b

BUSINESS CASUAL CAPSULE

9 + 5
8 + 4
3 + 11 + 5
4 + 9
4 + 11
5 + 8
6 + 8
6 + 9
6 + 11

CASUAL CAPSULE

10 + 1 + 7
10 + 5
12
12 + 6a
10 + 4
10 + 6
10 + 7 + 6a

For fabrics refer to pages 134–135.

FROM OFFICE TO EVENING

With so many woman working full time but still wanting to have a social life after work, here is how to adapt your business look to something you can go out in but still feel glamorous—without having to take a complete new outfit to work or going home to change.

THE STARTING POINTS

Make sure that normal body maintenance is up-to-date. If you know you have a date coming up in the diary, book your hairdresser, get your manicure (long-lasting is a good idea) and pedicure done, and make sure your makeup bag has all the essentials that you will need to complete your look.

Wear a garment during the day that can be adapted easily, though it will still need to be suitable for a day's work: so not sheer, low cut, too short, nor too tight!

One of the easiest items of clothing to dress up is the little black dress, but if black is not in your palette, choose an alternative color that is. If you work in a formal environment, make it navy or gray. If it is sleeveless make sure you have a jacket or cardigan you can wear over it. If dresses are not your scene, perhaps a really well-fitting pair of pants or skirt will be suitable for glamorizing.

The secret of this successful transition is in the accessories, which make something plain into something special. Accessories are best when teamed with plain garments. It takes a great deal of skill to successfully accessorize a floral or heavily patterned dress without it looking overdone!

ESSENTIALS

• Make sure you don't forget anything—write down a list the night before if necessary.

• Get up early and make sure you have time to do your hair properly and prepare your skin for your makeup.
• Two handbags: one large enough to carry all your evening glamour pieces to wear and a small jeweled or beaded bag or clutch that fits inside the larger one.
• Sheer or even fishnet stockings.
• A fun pair of glam shoes with high heels or flats to suit your style personality and occasion.
• Sparkling jewels for a glamorous evening.
• Don't forget your hair—sometimes just running your fingers through your hairstyle will be enough. If your hair is long, you may want to put it up and use an interesting hair accessory or pin.

THE MAKEOVER

Our model is wearing a simple black shift dress and jacket teamed with a plain pair of pumps and neutral stockings. Her handbag is large enough to take all her daytime and nighttime essentials.

At the end of a busy day our model starts by refreshing her makeup. Renew eyeliner, apply a deeper shade of eye shadow, and re-apply your mascara. Re-apply blush and apply a slightly brighter, stronger lip pencil and of course your lipstick.

Transformation complete: our model has changed her stockings to fishnet ones, removed her jacket and replaced it with a beautiful sheer scarf thrown over her shoulders. She changed her earrings and, finally, is carrying a pretty, detailed clutch.

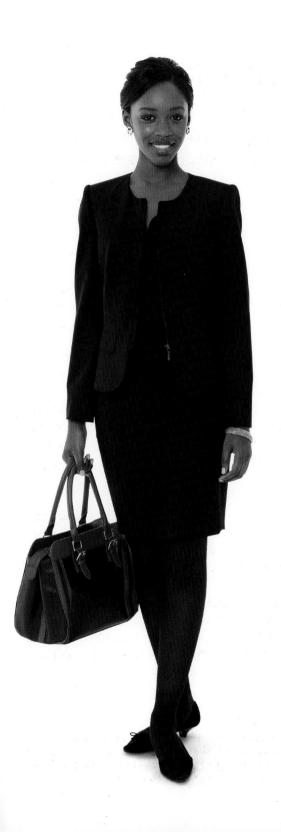
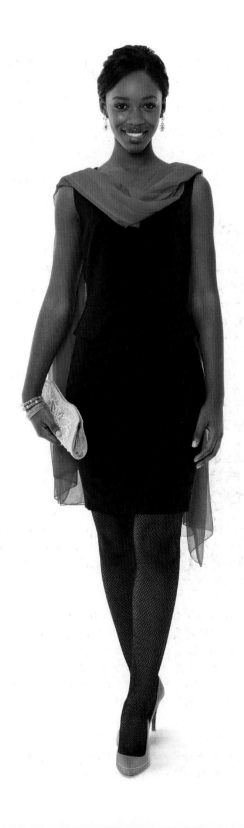

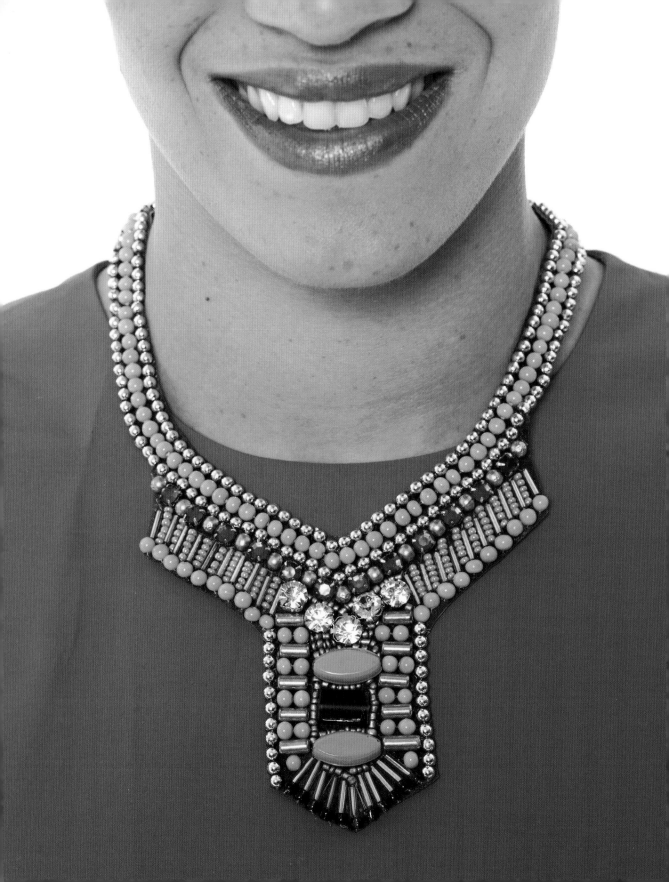

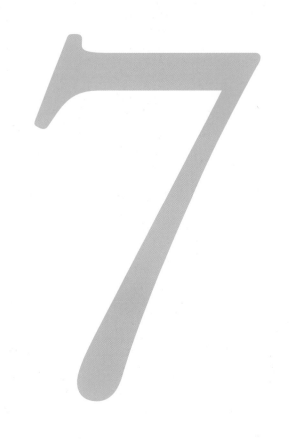

YOUR EVERYDAY
WARDROBE

UNDERWEAR

What you wear underneath your clothes is as important as your clothes themselves. Good foundation gives you support, a good all-over silhouette and will keep in check parts of your body that may need some holding back.

BRAS

A bra is an important investment, since it provides essential support for your breasts as well as creating the foundation for your outfit.

- Buy bras for different outfits and occasions: seamless, strapless, sports, and so on.
- Get measured professionally once a year and try on a range of styles from different brands—some cuts will fit you better than others.
- The back of your bra should sit comfortably in the middle of your back.
- Your breasts should not hang over the cups.
- If you have heavy breasts, a bra with nonstretch straps will be more supportive.
- If you have a fleshy back, three hooks are better than two.
- Fasten a new bra on the widest hooks and move inward as the bra stretches with wear.

Different styles of bras

There are many different styles and shapes of bra, and to get a smooth and well-shaped bust you need to choose the right style. Your choice of bra will depend on what you plan to wear on top of it. Most women will need two or three different styles in their lingerie drawer, depending on their shapes and lifestyle.

- **Bra top** This is where the cups are part of a T-shirt, and are suitable only for the small-chested.
- **T-shirt/seamless** This gives a cleaner line underneath tight clothing and lightweight fabrics.
- **Sports** This style will give good support to the bust and is designed to reduce breast bounce when exercising. It is also suitable to wear during pregnancy or when you are nursing.
- **Non-wired/soft** If you have a wide back it will be easier to find a better fit with a non-wired bra than one with an underwire. If you are having breast treatment surgery this is the recommended bra to wear until such time as you are fully recovered.
- **Underwire** This style offers added support and shape and minimizes sagging, and is the most versatile style for women.
- **Balconette** A low neckline that goes straight across the bust, with wide-set straps for a square neckline. These are suitable for wearing with lower cut tops.
- **Full cup bra** The entire breast is covered and the bra is designed to give full support.
- **Minimizer** This redistributes the breast so it does not protrude as much. These bras are good to wear under shirts. The advice for women with a larger bust, though, is to avoid wearing a front-opening shirt.
- **Push-up** This lifts the bust up and enhances the cleavage because it is padded. This style is not appropriate for the work environment.
- **Plunge bra** This is similar to a push-up bra but is unpadded. It suits a fuller bust because minimum coverage enables the cleavage to be exposed, creating the desired appearance under clothes.
- **Padded** These enhance a small bust and give it a slight lift. Some come with removable inserted pads.
- **Strapless bra** These bras are practical yet they are often complicated to fit. The back of a strapless bra must be firm enough to stay in place and for this reason, you may find you need a different size to your regular bra size.

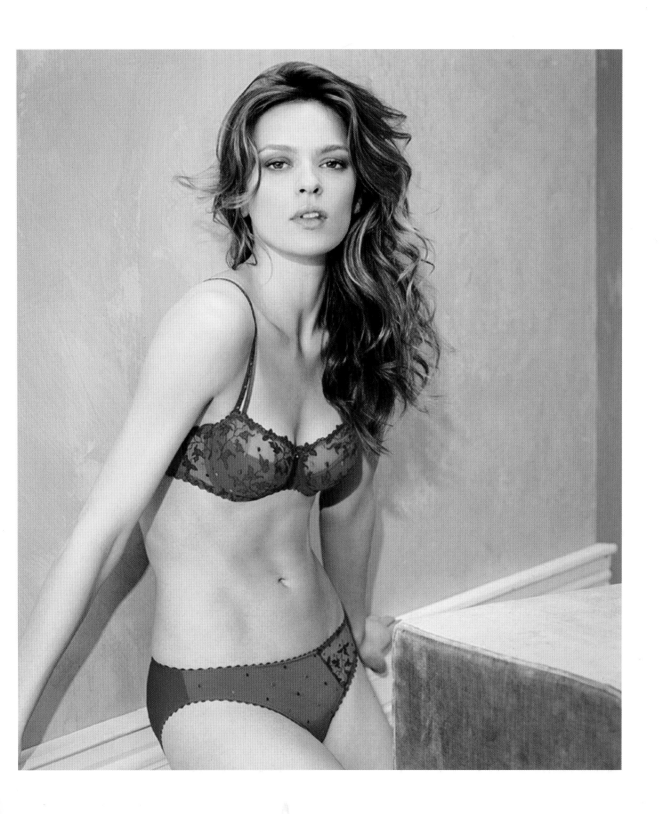

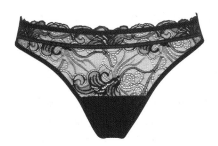

Thong/g-string

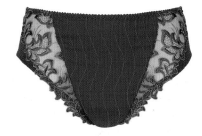

Deep brief

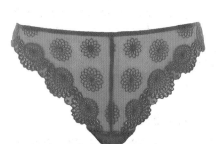

Bikini brief

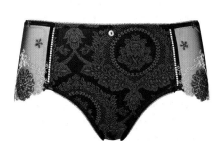

Tanga brief

Boyshorts/boxers

Hipster brief

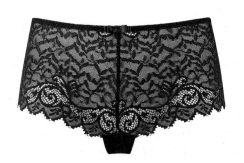

Tap pants

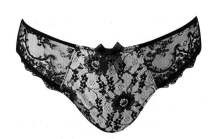

Italian brief

PANTIES

There is no excuse for VPLs (visible panty lines); with so much choice available, you should be able to find a cut and fit that's right for you.

- Buy bigger-sized panties than you think you will need. This will eliminate visible panty lines by ensuring that the elastic doesn't cut into your flesh. Panties are also notorious for shrinking in the wash.
- If you need tummy control, make sure the fit is good and that your flesh doesn't roll over the top when you sit down.

Different styles of panties

- **Thong/g-string** The traditional way to banish the VPL, which leaves the bottom bare. They are great for pants and fitted clothes, but are only suitable for those who are slim and/or who have pert bottoms.
- **Deep brief** The waistband sits on or just below the bellybutton and gives full side and back coverage. These are good for long bodies and hourglasses, and for bottoms that do not need any control.
- **Bikini and tanga briefs** These are shorter in the rise than the deep brief, but work for all body shapes.
- **Boyshorts/boxers** These have a lower-cut leg, which finishes at the top of the leg rather than across the bottom. Good against VPL and certainly more comfortable than thongs for larger bottoms. They are not good for rectangles.
- **Hipster brief** This is very short in the rise with little shape. Not suitable for women with a full tummy.
- **Tap pants** A comfortable, loose feminine cut with no control, which is perfect under full skirts and dresses. This knicker style is great for women with fuller hips and thighs.
- **Italian brief** This is good for people who are short in the rise, Inverted Triangles and Rectangles.

SHAPEWEAR

Shapewear is becoming more and more popular as fabric technology improves and the garments are becoming more comfortable to wear. However, it is not advisable to try and alter your body shape by encasing it in spandex.

- **Control tights** These offer the lightest control of all with the panty section of the tights offering an all-over control top for a little toning.
- **Tummy control** These come in different styles from brief to full shorts and have a control front panel in stretch fabric to shape and support the tummy.
- **Control panties** These offer support beneath clothing, and are designed specifically to offer a smooth and firm line under any clingy or close-fitting garment; control panties are ultimately seamless. They will be comfortable if the right size is purchased—don't be tempted to buy a smaller size to minimize your look.
- **Control bodies** These are specially designed to support the body throughout. The all-in-one shape to the body will support and enhance the bust, while flattening the stomach and firming the bottom. They are good when you want a smooth silhouette.
- **Waist nippers** These pull the waist in and create a waist under clothing.

STOCKINGS/PANTYHOSE

A woman used to be considered not properly dressed unless she wore stockings/pantyhose, whatever the weather. Nowadays, unless you work in a formal environment or are attending a formal event, it is usually acceptable to go without stockings/pantyhose in summer, as long as your legs are hair- and blemish-free. Always wear stockings/pantyhose with a business suit.

- Natural-colored stockings/pantyhose are suitable for most occasions.
- To elongate your legs, wear stockings/pantyhose that are the same color as your skirt or shoes.
- Balance the denier of your stockings/pantyhose with the fabric weight of your skirt or pants. In summer, with a lightweight fabric, seven to ten denier is ideal. In winter, with corduroy or tweed, you may consider opaques (30+ denier).
- Textured tights/pantyhose will give your outfit a fun twist, but they can add volume to the leg.

ACCESSORIES

Shoes and boots will update your look easily, so you should invest in at least one new pair every season. Bags and hats are also key items in creating your look and are a good way to reinforce your style personality. Belts are useful for balancing your proportions, but the style you choose and how you wear them will depend on your body shape. Scarves are a great way to introduce your colors.

BAGS

As well as carrying belongings, your handbag makes a style statement, and the bag you choose will be dictated by your style personality: go to pages 22–37. Like shoes, a bag can make or break your look, so here are some key pointers to help you choose:

- Different occasions call for different styles and sizes of handbag, so try to build up a collection that is appropriate for various occasions and outfits. Don't take a floral straw bag to a business meeting, nor a formal leather handbag to a dinner dance.
- Your bag needs to be in balance with your scale: a large bag will overwhelm a petite person, while a tiny bag will look lost on a grand-scale woman.
- The shape of your bag needs to follow the line of your body.
- Softer, unstructured bags work best for those with a Full Hourglass or Oval shape.
- Rectangles and Inverted Triangles need structured bags to reflect the lines and angles of their bodies.
- Triangles should avoid bags that hang at hip level, as they will add width to the widest area.
- Before you buy a handbag, look at yourself carrying it to check that it looks right for you.

FOOTWEAR

Like all accessories, the type of shoes or boots you wear can kill your look, so make sure they are appropriate for your outfit. Follow these guidelines:

- The height of heel you choose will often be determined by your comfort level, but a high or a narrow heel always adds length to the leg.
- If you are wearing a short skirt, a lower heel will make your legs look longer.
- Low-fronted shoes give the illusion of longer legs and narrower ankles; closed shoes shorten the length of the feet and legs.
- When choosing shoes with straps, bear in mind that low-cut T-straps work for most people, while ankle straps will only look good on those with long legs and slim ankles.
- When buying boots, check that the boot—whether ankle, calf-height, or full-length—stops at a narrow point on your legs.
- Sandals are ideal for vacations and hot weather, but your feet must be in immaculate condition. They should never be worn with business suits.
- Flat pumps are wonderful for anyone with average to long legs and thin ankles. Satin, velvet, or beaded pumps are good choices for evening, teamed with long skirts or pants.

SCARVES

Even if you don't own many clothes in your colors, a scarf is a great way to experiment and instantly gives you the right shade near your face.

- Skinny scarves will look out of proportion on grand-scale women.

- Petite women should avoid oversized scarves, such as full-size pashminas, as these can swamp your appearance.
- Do not tie scarves under your chin if you have a short neck.
- A long, thin scarf draped around your neck will make your body appear longer and slimmer.

BELTS

Belts are great fashion accessories that can update your look. Worn cleverly, belts can also help to balance the proportions of your upper and lower body and define the waist.

- You need a waist to wear a belt, so they are not ideal for Rectangles or Oval body shapes.
- Narrow and lightweight belts are best on petite to average women.
- Wide, statement belts are best on average to long-bodied women.
- Belts must work with the rest of your look.

JEWELRY

If making a statement, just wear one piece so that you don't overpower your look; otherwise your jewelry should balance with your scale.

HATS

Hats date quickly and won't necessarily have much longevity in your wardrobe. However, they can turn a plain outfit into something special.

- Brims should not extend beyond your shoulders.
- Grand-scale women should avoid pill-box hats, which will look out of proportion.
- Petite women should not be tempted by large, wide-brimmed hats.
- Complement your face with your hat shape. Rounded crowns, and brims in loosely woven straw or soft fabrics suit round faces.
- Square or rectangular faces will look good in flat crowns and straight brims.

- A downward-sloping brim doesn't work with a short neck, and can emphasize jowls; a brim with an upward tilt will help to lift the face.
- A completely coordinated outfit with matching hat looks contrived; a complementary or contrasting color adds interest to an outfit.
- Dark colors cast a shadow over your face.

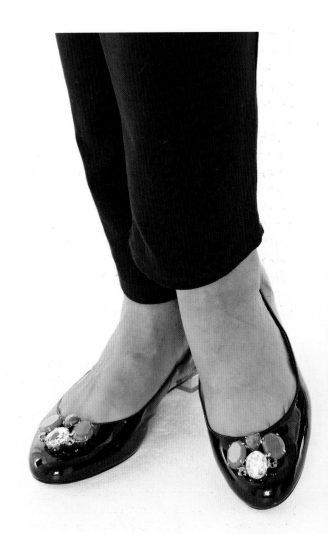

ORGANIZING YOUR CLOSET

Now that you've established your colors, style personality, and body shape, and seen how to pull a look together, you have to make it all work for you. Start at the place where you keep most of your clothes: your closet.

CLOSET AUDIT

The best way to check out what you have, what works and what doesn't work in your closet is to go through each item of clothing piece by piece. You will end up with three piles:
- **Pile 1**: Clothes you will keep
- **Pile 2**: Clothes you might keep
- **Pile 3**: Clothes that must go

How you decide

- Is it the right color? If the answer is yes, then ask yourself if it is the right style? If it is, it goes in pile 1.
- If it's the right color but the wrong style, can it be altered or worn differently to make it work? If it can, it goes in pile 2.
- Is it the right style but the wrong color? Can you wear it with a complementary color from your palette? Do you have a scarf in a color that will make it work? If yes, it goes in pile 2.
- If it's the wrong color and the wrong style, it goes in pile 3.
- If it's not your current size and you haven't worn it for a year, it goes in pile 3.

Pile 1 – Clothes for keeps

- Organize garments by categories: coats, jackets, suits, skirts, pants, dresses, blouses, and shirts. Grouping by color within these categories will give you ideas for combining clothes.
- Button up jackets and coats, and pull up zippers, so that garments hang straight before you put them in the closet, all facing the same way.

- Don't put anything back in the closet unless it's clean.
- Don't overcrowd your closet.

Pile 2 – Is it worth keeping?

- Check every piece against what you have in your closet to see whether it is worth keeping.
  You might find that a jacket in the wrong color, for example, can be made to work for you if worn with a top that you've decided to keep.
- Shortening the hem will salvage a skirt that's too long.
- Changing the buttons on a jacket will give it a new lease of life.

Pile 3 – Dispose of clothes as you see fit

- Give them to a friend.
- Sell expensive items and those that are still current and of good quality.
- Donate them to a thrift store.

Finishing touches

Before you put everything back in your closet, vacuum and dust it, and place some moth-repellent products at the bottom. To preserve the shape of your clothes, you will need the correct hangers.
- Sturdy wooden hangers for jackets and coats.
- Wooden hangers with clips for skirts and pants.
- Padded or non-slip hangers for lightweight and delicate, luxury fabrics.
- Basic plastic hangers for blouses, shirts, and lightweight summer dresses.

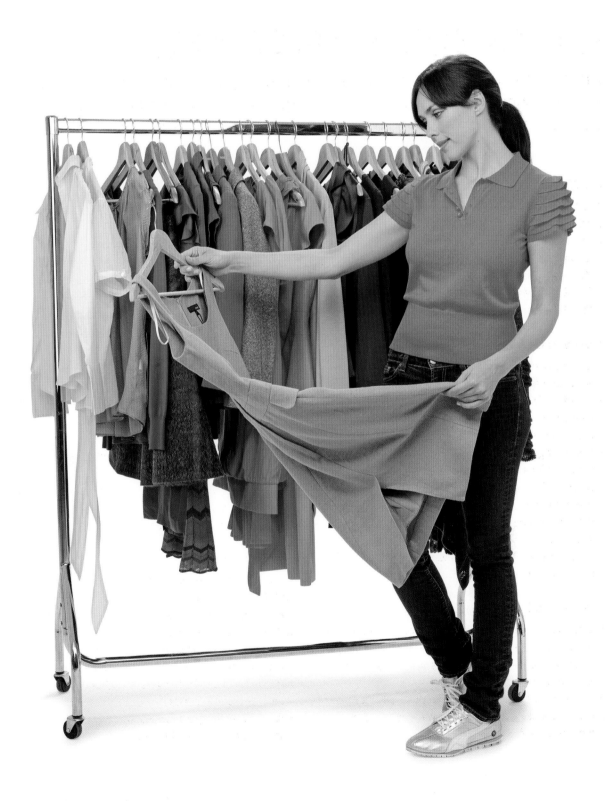

LOOKING BEAUTIFUL WITH A BUMP

Being pregnant will give most women some new challenges in the wardrobe department. Your body shape and weight will alter over the months and there will be emotional highs and lows due to all the hormone changes taking place. To feel confident during this exciting time, a little thought for what you choose to wear will make this a more pleasurable experience.

THE MONTHS AHEAD

- During your pregnancy, your proportions will not change, although your waist definition will go. So the general rules on proportions will remain the same: go to pages 136–137.
- To ensure that pregnancy doesn't take a toll on your bust, it is important to be fitted regularly for a bra over the coming months, as your bust size will definitely increase.
- There will be times when your energy levels will sink; color will give you the boost that you need, as well as making you look healthier and fitter. For more on this see Chapter 3, pages 38–49.

EARLY DAYS

Your bust starts enlarging and your waist begins to thicken, but you can fit into your "normal" clothes.

- Check out your wardrobe for shirts, cardigans, empire-style dresses, and tops that will accommodate these changes.
- Pants and skirts can be left undone a little, as long as this doesn't alter the way they hang.
- Shorter dresses and tunics look great over leggings, or over jeans and pants in which you may not be able to do the waist up.
- As much as you may be tempted to wear your partner's baggy sweatpants, this is to be avoided at all costs!

BLOOMING DAYS

You will now start telling the world about your forthcoming event. However, this doesn't mean you have to wear a tent! You need to purchase a few key pieces that will take you through the coming months and that you can accessorize for fun and color. If buying specially designed maternity clothes, stick to your "normal" size. Small and petite women may find it easier to buy one or two sizes larger in standard clothing and then shorten the garments.

Pants

Your first stop should be to find the best fitting pants and/or jeans that will accommodate your expanding bump.

Dresses

Dresses will be a longer-lasting option than skirts. Wrap and empire-styles are perfect and fabric with some stretch will gently skim your bump.

Tops

How you show off your bump is very much a personal choice. Some women like a tight-fitting look that shows off their natural shape plus bump; others will feel more comfortable in a looser, more fluid garment that discreetly shows their increasing bump.

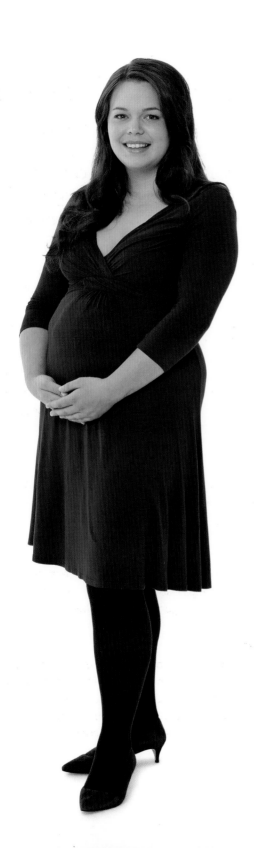

Shoes

Your high heels and favorite fashion shoes will need a rest until the baby is born because the extra weight you will be carrying may make your feet wider and you may wobble on those elegant heels. You can still remain fashionable wearing some well-constructed flats or wedge shoes. Flat pumps are pretty but do not give you the support you need—only wear them occasionally. Get measured properly to ensure your shoes give you good support.

Accessories

Your "normal" accessories will still work and enhance your look. If you miss shopping trips, a new pair of earrings or a new handbag can still give you the boost you need. Remember to balance the proportion of your bump with the size of your bag! Thinking ahead, you will need a larger bag for all the baby paraphernalia—and that's a wonderful excuse for a new bag.

NEARLY THERE

Pamper yourself in these later weeks—there won't be time once the baby arrives.

You can still look glamorous and feminine, and don't forsake prettiness for practicality. Have a mani-pedi, keep up your skincare and makeup routine, and discuss with your hairdresser a low-maintenance hairstyle for the months to come.

Rings can get tight in the last few weeks and you may want to store them until you can slip them back on again—buy some fun costume jewelry instead.

GLAMOROUS OCCASIONS

It's so exciting to get an invitation to a special occasion, be it a wedding, a family celebration, or a special night out with a new date. Choosing an outfit that is current, but not high fashion, will ensure the longevity of the clothes—that asymmetric shoulder line will look out of place in a year's time. A simple dress with the right accessories will be timeless.

YOUR STYLE PERSONALITY

"Glamming up" will mean different things to different women. This is where understanding your style personality will come into its own: go to pages 24–25. Some of you may like to just get the investment jewelry out, while others will rush to the mall and buy the latest trends.

Creative

You will have a ball dreaming up something different to wear. Vintage clothes will be a great choice. Try something lacy and don't forget the antique jewelry and perhaps a beaded bag. In colder weather, go for velvets and velours, and even fake fur. For more Creative style ideas, go to pages 26–27.

Dramatic

You will definitely want a completely new outfit, but before you rush out, go through your closet and see what is lurking there. Maybe just a new pair of colorful shoes or a new top will give you the wow factor. For more Dramatic style ideas, go to pages 28–29.

Romantic

You are in your element. You are bound to have something pretty already in your wardrobe, but make sure it is appropriate for the event. If you'll be standing for a long time, you may have to sacrifice the killer heels for a more comfortable pair. Don't forget to book all your pampering treatments ahead of time so that you will really feel glamorous on the day. For more Romantic style ideas, go to pages 30–31.

Classic

If the event is a formal one, you will wear a suit with coordinated accessories; you may find a less-formal event a little more challenging. A dress with a complementary pashmina, shrug, or cardigan will be a good alternative. Don't forget to add a little sparkle, even if it is costume jewelry. Forget the flats and go for heeled sandals or peep-toe wedges. For more Classic style ideas, go to pages 32–33.

Natural

This is your least-favorite scenario, so keep it simple and comfortable. Go for a pantsuit for the formal occasion or a long skirt or pants for a more relaxed do. Don't forget grooming to show that you have made an effort. Don't feel shy about adding some jewelry; a simple strand of beads looks pretty without being fussy. Your best handbag choice will be one with a long strap. For more Natural style ideas, go to pages 34–35.

City chic

Your style of clothes will remain the same, but this time the fabrics will be more luxurious: think silks and satins. Add color to your usual neutrals with a scarf or shawl, some stunning jewelry, a dressy handbag, and a fun pair of shoes. For more City Chic style ideas, go to pages 36–37.

FINISHING TOUCHES

Now is the perfect opportunity to indulge in a little pampering and glamorize your hairstyle and makeup. There is nothing like a good haircut, color and a blow-dry to make you feel like a million dollars. You may even consider adding some sparkling clips or detailed headbands to your finished hairstyle. Allow plenty of time to apply your makeup and maybe go for a more vibrant or darker lipstick than you would normally wear. A dusting of shimmer anywhere on the face is flattering and glamorous, and a light spray of perfume will complete your outfit.

UNDERWEAR

Often your chosen outfit does not work with your normal, everyday lingerie. Thin straps, low backs and strapless dresses call for special underwear that will still give you the right support and shape, but without unsightly straps on show—there is nothing more embarrassing than, halfway through an event, your bra strap appearing or, worse still, your strapless top beginning to slip.

DRESSING FOR THE OCCASION
Make sure that you wear what is appropriate for the event. You do not want to outdo the hostess or be the only guest who has not made an effort. If in doubt, ask the host for guidelines on the dress code. To help you pull the look together, we suggest you find out about:

• The venue: inside or out
• The event: formal or informal
• The time: day or evening

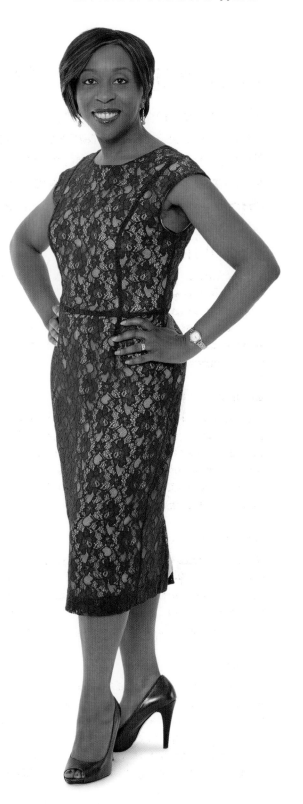

KEEPING CURRENT

As previously mentioned, fashion trends for women tend to go in five-year cycles, so keeping current and updating your look can take years off your image. Even though your clothes may still be in good condition, if the style is no longer in fashion, you should think of evolving, along with everything else.

WHAT TO CONSIDER

All aspects of your look need to be appraised on a regular basis: that means your hairstyle, makeup, clothes, shoes, and accessories.

Hairstyle

Think about the last time your changed your style. If it has been the same for more than five years it may be time to take a fresh look at it. Sometimes it might mean adjusting the color to one that is age-appropriate or changing the style to something that is more up-to-date. Do you still want long hair? Would a new hair cut give you a new lease of life? If your hairdresser doesn't think it needs a change and you do, then maybe it is time to change your hair stylist?

Makeup colors

We often say we can carbon date someone by the way they apply their makeup. Fashion colors change and so does the emphasis on how makeup is applied. Some years it is all about eyes, in others lipstick and gloss take the lead. Look around at cosmetic counters and see what they are promoting that season, or check out what your favorite magazine is advising. Once again, if you have been wearing the same color lipstick for years, it may be time you changed shades.

Clothes

It is always hard to dispose of any garment that still fits you but is out of fashion. The wise purchases, or investments buys, should be garments that do not date. The classic trench coat, for example, has not changed style or shape for years, which is why certain classic labels remain so popular. A classic pair of pants, or a good plain-colored skirt in one of your best neutrals will last for many years. If you love fashion, make your fashion buys fun, but do not necessarily invest heavily in them—they should be the fun-colored disposable items in your wardrobe.

Shoes

The height of the heel and the shape of the toe reveal whether a style of shoe is still in fashion or not. Extreme styles such as the gladiator sandal or high-platform shoe quickly date, but a pair of loafers or a classic mid-heel pump should last longer in your wardrobe. When you buy fashion shoes, wear them—they will date more quickly than any other item in your closet.

Accessories

Have fun with your accessories, they are an instant way to update your look and can be at any price range depending on your budget. Consider trends, for example the silk square versus the long pashmina. Costume jewelry will have trends too: the choker-style necklaces or long strings of beads. Whichever you choose, you need to consider your style personality, your scale, and proportions. You can always mix your investment pieces of jewelry with fashion items as long as they work together in scale and size. Don't forget that your handbag can date too.

By styling her hair, shortening the hemline, and adding up-to-date accessories, our model appears younger and slimmer.

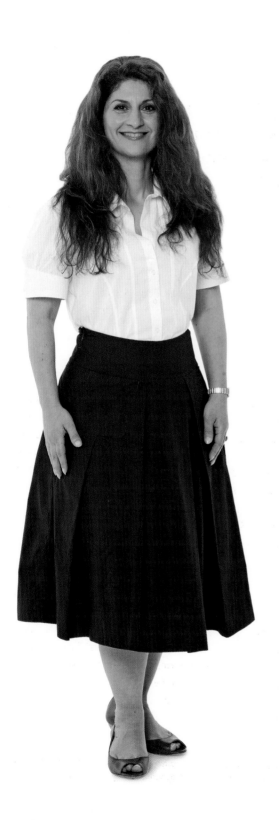
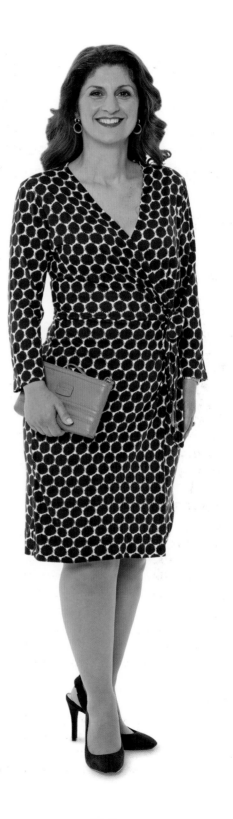

AGES & STAGES

Nothing dates a woman as much as wearing the same makeup at 50 as she did when she was 25—your style of makeup and the way you apply it should change as you mature. A good skincare regime and a healthy lifestyle, together with the right clothes, colors, and style, are essential for looking good and feeling confident. Here are a few winning tips to help you evolve your look as you mature.

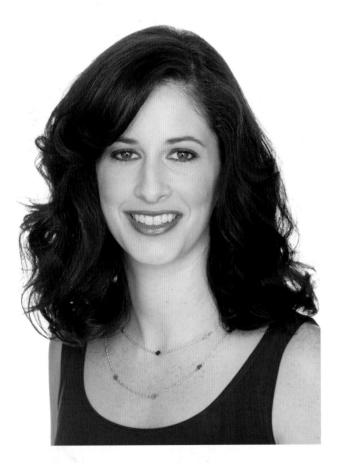

A good skincare regime and a healthy lifestyle will keep you looking and feeling good

WHEN YOU ARE 30–40

- You should have established a good skincare routine: cleansing, toning, and moisturizing every single day; exfoliating and applying a treatment mask appropriate to your skin type—dry, oily, sensitive, or normal—once a week.
- Ensure that you are using high-factor sunblocks year-round to protect your skin from harmful UVB rays and aging UVA rays.
- Learn to recognize good-quality cosmetic products that offer the most benefits.
- Wearing foundation every day will protect your skin.
- You are no longer a teenager, so makeup with glitter and sparkle should only be worn for parties, and even then in moderation.
- High-fashion makeup looks are for the runway models only.
- Make regular appointments with a dental hygienist to ensure that you have a dazzling smile.

WHEN YOU ARE 40–50

- Keep positive when the first gray hairs and lines start to appear.
- Throw away frosted eye shadows, glossy lipsticks, and colored mascaras. Don't overdo the fake tan and avoid orangey shades.
- Feed and nourish your skin regularly.

- Keep to a simple makeup routine. Apply a minimum of base (foundation or tinted moisturizer and concealer as needed), blusher, mascara, and lipstick.

- Don't be afraid to use a little powder to create a more groomed look, but be careful not to apply too much and make sure you blend it well, because it can collect in and draw attention to fine lines.

- Use blushers and bronzers to emphasize facial bone structure and add definition to your face, particularly if you're carrying a little extra weight here.

WHEN YOU ARE 50+

- Indulge yourself with the occasional pampering treat at a spa or beauty salon.

- A skincare regime is a must. Now is the time to use products that have been specially formulated for mature skins.

- Keep abreast of the latest beauty technology so that you can benefit from new products.

- Don't forget the rest of your body. Use a skin-firming body moisturizer morning and night, and always after bathing.

- Pay special attention to your décolletage—smooth face cream downward and body cream upward.

- Your beauty routine will now include paying more attention to your eyebrows. As well as grooming they may need to be enhanced either with an eyebrow pencil or a regular tinting.

- Less is more when it comes to makeup.

- An eye base is now essential, as it will prevent your lids from looking creased when wearing eye shadow.

- A lip base will help to prevent lipstick from bleeding and avoid a "buttonhole" lip.

- Use powder on the bony parts of your face only, and avoid the soft, fleshy areas, such as eyelids and the area just below the eyes.

- Keep up regular visits to the dentist and hygienist.

- Watch out for and remove any stray whiskers that might start to appear.

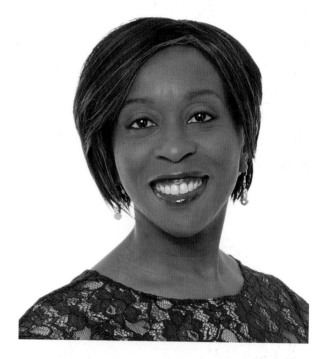

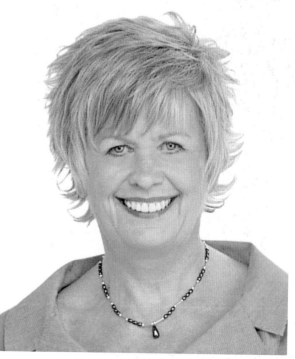

HOW TO SHOP

Inevitably, in the course of organizing your closet, you will dispose of items that need to be replaced in colors and styles that suit you. To help you in this next phase, make a list of what you need to complete your wardrobe.

INVESTMENT BUYS

It's not the cost of an investment buy that matters, rather it's how often you wear it. A bargain garment that you wear only once is a costly purchase compared to an expensive item that you wear a hundred times. Investment pieces will vary according to your lifestyle and personality, but they will consist of overcoats, jackets, skirts, dresses, and pants.

FASHION BUYS

These are the items that you buy every year to keep your core wardrobe updated and that are fun to wear. They could be anything from a current color or the latest style in tops or dresses.

IT'S THE FIT THAT COUNTS

• Sizes will vary depending on where you shop and the cut of the item.
• The looser the fit, the slimmer you look—and you'll undoubtedly feel more comfortable.

ACHIEVING AN ELEGANTLY LOOSE FIT

• You should be able to fit a finger underneath a waistband.
• Side seams should hang straight with no horizontal creases, especially on hips and thighs.
• Zippers should lie flat.
• Allow some give in the sleeve around the upper arm.
• Skirts and pants should hang straight from the buttocks and not curve under.
• Sleeves on jackets and coats should finish at the wrist.
• Pockets shouldn't gape.

• There should be no pulling around the bust on jackets, blouses, or dresses.

RECOGNIZING QUALITY

• Seams should lie flat and not pull or wrinkle.
• Hemlines should be flat and even.
• Linings or facings must lie flat and not show.
• An expensive price tag doesn't always mean a quality finish.
• Buttonholes should not have loose threads.

SHOPPING TIPS

• Make a list, but don't be over-ambitious about how much you can achieve in one trip.
• Wear appropriate underwear.
• Take with you the shoes that you'll be wearing with the garment you're buying.
• Look first for the right color: refer to pages 52–111; then ensure that the style suits your body shape, proportions, and scale: go to pages 122–151; and, finally, your style personality: go to pages 24–37.
• Take only three or four pieces at a time into the changing room.
• Make sure the item fits and feels comfortable.
• Do you like yourself in it?
• If it's over your budget, is it really worth it?
• Beware the over-enthusiastic sales assistant.

KEEPING IT LOOKING GOOD

• Clothes that crease easily, such as linens, need laundering after each wearing.
• Tailored suits need to be hung up for them to air.

- Shoes absorb moisture when they're worn, which needs to evaporate before you wear them another day.
- Keep dry-cleaning to a minimum, as the fluids will damage and weaken the fibers.
- Repair any damage to your clothes (loose hems, missing buttons, or snags) immediately.
- Clean your shoes regularly, and use shoe trees.

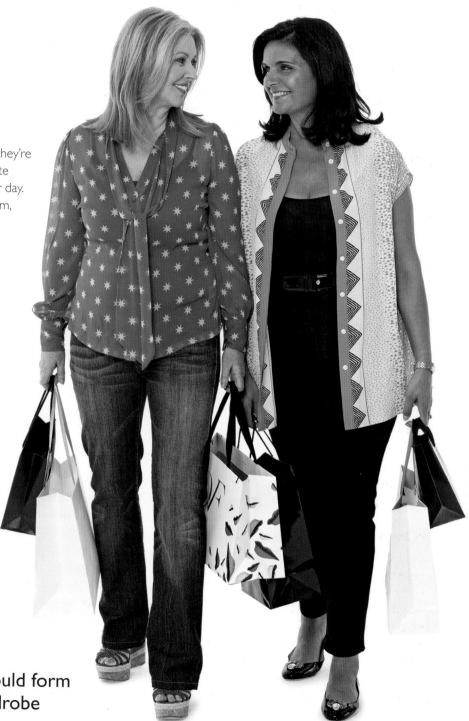

Investment pieces should form the core of your wardrobe

PERFECT PACKING

Most women return from vacation with a suitcase of clothes they haven't worn. With airlines today charging more and more for checked luggage, learning to pack light is the order of the day, and by taking hand luggage only, think of the extra time you'll save when you arrive at your destination.

PACKING RULES

- Pack as few clothes as possible.
- Wear your heavier shoes/boots/coat.
- Decant your toiletries into travel-sized plastic bottles.
- Minimize your makeup bag—you don't need 10 lipsticks and eye shadows.
- Wear your valuable jewelry and keep the costume jewelry light.
- One perfume only.
- Don't go over the top with underwear—it can be washed overnight.
- Ensure that your traveling handbag is large enough to carry your documents and other essentials, and put a pouch inside it that will be able to double up as an evening bag.

YOUR TRAVELING WARDROBE

List out every day of your trip, and for each day write down what you might be doing (lunch, sightseeing, sporting activity, or just relaxing). For each of these, make a note of what you are likely to wear. This will demonstrate that indeed you can wear the same pair of pants twice, and therefore how little you need to pack.

- Following your list, lay all the clothes out on the bed, and see how they coordinate with each other. There is no point in taking the little red sparkly top "just in case" if you do not pack something to go with it.
- Keep the colors you take to a minimum. Your pants and jacket should be in neutral shades, which will work with everything else.

- If you have forgotten something, have fun and buy it locally! You need to leave some space in your suitcase for anything you may want to bring back.

On the next page are some basic packing guidelines to make your planning easier.

Bon voyage!

THE CITY BREAK (3 days/2 nights)

- 1 waterproof jacket/coat
- 1 versatile, neutral jacket that you can glamorize
- 1 pair of pants
- 1 pair of jeans

- 1 dress
- 1 skirt
- 1 twin-set (top + cardigan)
- 1 shirt/blouse
- 1 T-shirt

- 1 pashmina
- 1 pair of loafers/comfortable shoes
- 1 pair of heels
- underwear for 3 days + 1 spare (in case of delay)

DAY	DAYTIME	EVENING
1 Travel	Jacket, pants, top (from twin-set), loafers	Jacket, dress, heels
2	Jeans, T-shirt, waterproof/jacket, loafers	Skirt, blouse, heels, pashmina
3	Pants, twin-set, loafers	Dress, cardigan (from twin-set), heels
Travel home	Jeans, blouse, jacket, loafers	

THE ONE WEEK BEACH VACATION

- 1 pair of jeans
- 1 pair of cropped pants
- 1 pair of shorts
- 2 dresses
- 1 skirt
- 1 caftan
- 1 fancy T-shirt

- 3 T-shirts
- 1 cotton twin-set (strappy top + cardigan)
- 1 pair of sneaker-style shoes
- 1 pair of pretty sandals or flip flops
- 1 pair of heels
- 1 pair of ballet shoes

- 1 pashmina
- 3 bathing suits/bikinis
- 1 hat
- underwear for 4 days (do a wash every other day)
- your travel bag will double up as a beach bag!

DAY	AM/PM	EVENING
1 Travel	Jeans, twin-set, sneaker-style shoes	Cropped pants, fancy T-shirt, pretty sandals
2 Beach	Shorts, T-shirt 1, sandals/flip flops	Dress 1, heels, pashmina
3 Pool	Caftan, sandals/flip flops	Skirt, strappy top, ballet shoes
4 Beach	Shorts, T-shirt 2, sandals/flip flops	Dress 2, heels
5 Sightseeing	Cropped pants, T-shirt 1, sneaker-style shoes	Skirt, fancy T-shirt, ballet shoes
6 Beach	Shorts, T-shirt 3, sandals/flip flops	Dress 1, heels
7 Pool	Caftan, sandals	Dress 2 or new dress bought locally, heels
Travel home	Jeans, T-shirt 2, cardigan (from twin-set)	

INDEX

ACKNOWLEDGMENTS

AUTHOR ACKNOWLEDGMENTS

When we first started putting down on paper all that we, and our stylish image consultants, knew in 2006 for *Color Me Confident*, little did we know that in 2010 this particular book would be revisited—and now here we are in 2014, and we are onto our third edition. So a huge thank you to everyone who has bought the book in one of its editions and helped to make it the bestseller that it is the world over.

For this edition we have added lots more examples of models with different types of coloring, and we hope that you will recognize yourself in one of the photographs. Of course, there is no quick-and-easy rule to figure out where you fit in within the parameters of this book as we are all individuals and what **colour me beautiful** do is an art (with some science thrown in for good measure). If you don't find yourself in this book, may we respectfully suggest that you find an image consultant/stylist who can help you.

We have had tremendous support from the Hamlyn team—this is their book as much as ours. Particular thanks go to Stephanie Jackson, Clare Churly, Jennifer Veall, Lucy Carter, and the designer with the flair, Yasia Williams-Leedham.

No illustrated book would be complete without models. Some of them are professionals, others are our consultants and friends, who each brought with them their own style and their clothes too. They are: Alia Al Monla, Jacqui Cooper, Anna de Vere, Kathy Ennis, Audrey Hanna, Ivy Rose Harris, Mandy Lehto, Jo Moir, Ann Skidmore, Mary Stewart, Rachel Watson, and Liz Willetts. Without our models this book would not be such a happy and smiling one. Thank you for being so real, so gorgeous, so enthusiastic, and so patient in front of Ruth Jenkinson's camera. Grateful thanks to Victoria Barnes and her team at the hair and makeup stations. There were 12 of us on the shoot before the models arrived—and we are all still great friends—it was the best team ever.

Special thanks to the following companies who lent us so many garments, shoes and handbags:

- box2.co.uk
- kettlewellcolours.co.uk
- lkbennett.com
- radley.co.uk
- rigbyandpeller
- spiritoftheandes.co.uk
- wall-london.com

And thank you to the lovely Nikki Ahmed (nicolaahmed.com) for sourcing so many more of everything than was needed.

We have now worked together for 25 years and we still love working together, we love what we do, and we love sharing it all with you.

Pat and Veronique

For more information on services, products and how to become a consultant go to www.colourmebeautiful.co.uk

66 the business centre
15–17 Ingate Place
London SW3 5LN
info@colourmebeautiful.co.uk
t: +44(0)20 7627 5211

PICTURE ACKNOWLEDGMENTS

All photographs are by Ruth Jenkinson for Octopus Publishing with the exception of the following:

Corbis Rolf Haid/dpa 53 above right.

Getty Images David Mepham/FilmMagic 27; Don Arnold/ WireImage 73 above right; Francois Durand 83; Frazer Harrison 82; Gregg DeGuire/WireImage 103 above left; James Devaney/WireImage 73 above left; Jason LaVeris/Film-Magic 93 above left; Jon Kopaloff/FilmMagic 72; Mark Metcalfe 53 above left; NBCU Photo Bank via Getty Images 29; Sasha Mordovets 33; Valerie Macon 83 above right; Vittorio Zunino Celotto 63 above right.

Rex 118; Agencia EFE 31; BDG 37; Broadimage 62; Farr/ Schneider Press/SIPA 92; Matt Baron/BEI 63 above left; MediaPunch 102; Startraks Photo 35, 52, 93 above right, 103 above right.

Publishing Director: Stephanie Jackson
Managing Editor: Clare Churly
Deputy Art Director: Yasia Williams-Leedham
Picture Library Manager: Jennifer Veall
Photographer: Ruth Jenkinson
Hair and Make-up Artists: Victoria Barnes, Simone Vollmer, and Roisin Donaghy
Stylist: Nikki Ahmed
Models from MOT Models, Hughes Models, Source Models, and ModelPlan
Illustrators: Jill Bay and Abigail Read
Assistant Production Manager: Lucy Carter